CONTENTS

FOREWORD BY NEIL BACK AND ALAN PEARSON

Rugby Union is a game of technical skill and tactical knowledge and underpinning this even more so today than ever before is physicality. To perform optimally players must train their aerobic and anaerobic fitness but at the business end it is all about strength, power and speed. Making tackles, controlling rucks, getting over the gain line are essential elements of the game and of course these are largely governed by your ability to exert greater strength, speed and power than your opponent.

I remember during the Rugby World Cup 2003 Semi-final battle versus the French that our teams conditioning, particularly our speed and power gave us the vital edge to secure victory and to go on to claim the ultimate prize versus Australia in the Final.

Having worked closely with Glen I can assure you that he is up there with the very best in the world. His knowledge, attention to detail and understanding of what is required to attain and sustain elite peak performance, especially with respect to speed and power, is second to none.

This book is a great introduction for developing your own speed and power. Glen has a first class understanding of being '*ready to train*' for optimum performance with plenty of detail on conditioning the body for strength prior to plyometric training. This is something usually overlooked by coaches and athletes which unfortunately leads to increases in injuries. In my opinion plyometrics should always be a part of any training programme where the end goal is increased speed and power and with it this book should be an essential tool in any athlete's or coach's library.

Neil Back MBE

Glen has been a Master SAQ Trainer for many years. His knowledge and practical application, passion and commitment to functional training is second to none. This book demonstrates his understanding of how best to prepare athletes using intensely researched best practice gathered from years of experience and knowledge. I highly recommend this book to all those who want improve physical performance.

Alan Pearson SAQ International

Plyometrics

FOR SPEED AND POWER

GLEN THURGOOD

Forewords by Neil Back MBE & Alan Pearson

THE CROWOOD PRESS

First published in 2016 by
The Crowood Press Ltd
Ramsbury, Marlborough
Wiltshire SN8 2HR

www.crowood.com

© Glen Thurgood 2016

British Library Cataloguing-in-Publication Data
A catalogue record for this book is available from the British Library.

ISBN 978 1 78500 041 6

Typeset by Servis Filmsetting Ltd, Stockport, Cheshire
Printed and bound in Malaysia by Times Offset (M) Sdn Bhd

ACKNOWLEDGEMENTS

The author and publishers would like to thank the following people and organizations for their generous help in producing this book. For modelling: Training Shed coaches Ryan Bates, Jack Campbell, Ethan Draycott, Will Gooch, Lydia Palmer, Jack Young; for use of facilities: Phil Littlewood (Training Shed Market Harborough), Jack Young and Will Gooch (Training Shed Stratford-upon-Avon); for use of equipment: Alan Pearson (SAQ International); Jamie Taylor, Phil Littlewood (Indigo Fitness); photography: Ricky White (www.rickywhite.com).

This book has been made possible by the kind collaboration of the following companies.

TRAINING SHED

At the Training Shed we pride ourselves on offering first class facilities, twinned with the finest training and treatment services, that are not the norm in other gyms. As fitness professionals we have spent many years in the industry as coaches, personal trainers, physiotherapists, sports therapists and athletes, writing worldwide industry leading books and courses. We understand the importance of being fit for function. Whatever your aspirations or requirements we can offer a type of training or therapy to suit your needs. (www.trainingshed.com)

INDIGO FITNESS

Indigo Fitness has been at the forefront of performance strength training for almost twenty years, leading the market with innovative design, state of the art engineering and high quality equipment. We manufacture much of our equipment at our factory right here in the UK and are also UK exclusive distributors for Powerbag, Duraflex premium flooring and RAZE strength and conditioning equipment. (www.indigofitness.com)

SAQ INTERNATIONAL

SAQ International is a world leader in the benefits of human movement. SAQ provides training, education, consultancy and specialized equipment to elite sport clubs and individuals, NGBs, education and public health including early years fundamental movement and community physical activity programmes developed to improve health, well-being and education. During the past twenty years SAQ International has led the way in the practical application of ground-breaking movement-based programmes into all areas of sport and physical activity in many parts of the world. (www.saqinternational.com)

ABOUT THE AUTHOR

Glen Thurgood is a coach, physical therapist, author, speaker and athlete. Glen received his Masters in Strength and Conditioning from Coventry University in 2010. He is co-owner of Training Shed a functional training and performance facility in Market Harborough with two additional facilities and growing...

With over eighteen years experience both as an elite level performance coach and athlete, his wealth of knowledge and experience has led him to work with some of the world's leading coaches in both rugby and football. He has a huge passion for developing young athletes and has worked with many schools and national level academies. Glen also works with runners, triathletes, ironman athletes, martial arts, canoeists and cyclists.

1 | PLYOMETRICS – THE BEGINNING

Every good coach or athlete asks more questions than they answer. So before you set out on your quest for greater speed and power through the use of plyometrics, I would imagine you are wondering how it came into existence as a training modality. You don't need to read this bit to be more powerful or faster but, as a coach, I believe it is always good to know how something responsible for a monumental change in training methods evolved. Everything begins somewhere and with regards to the evolution of plyometrics as we know it today – it started in Russia with a high jumper.

Vladimir Dyachkov was that high jumper. Dyachkov was a great jumps athlete and won the Soviet high jump and pole vault title eleven times during the 1930s. After his career he went on to coach and was appointed national coach to the Soviet team and later head coach during the 1960, 1964 and 1968 Olympic Games. A studious coach, he amassed a wealth of knowledge by studying numerous films of the world's best high jumpers during the 1940s and 1950s. Dyachkov spent hours on end meticulously analyzing the footage, which led him to recognize a pattern in the technique of the better jumpers. He noticed that, just before take-off, it was the simple arm jumping

mechanics that improved overall jump height. Simply moving the arms into a backward position during the last step of the approach to the bar and then driving them forward and upward increased the drive of the take-off phase and, as a result, an increased high point at take-off. The technique during this period was the dive straddle technique – the current Fosbury Flop did not come into existence until Dick Fosbury won the 1968 Mexico Olympics. Dyachkov's observations of the straddle technique led him to develop new training methods for his high jump athletes and, of course, this new studious evidence-based approach to training led to success. Dyachkov's new coaching methods helped Soviet athlete Yuri Stepanov to high jump world record glory in 1957, setting the bar to a new height of 2.16m. This was an increase of 1cm but, probably more importantly for the Soviet Union, it broke a record previously held by Charles Dumas of the United States of America.

However, the new Soviet world record was controversial to say the least and not just because it showed Eastern dominance over the West. These days, if a record is broken the first question would be: 'And what was the result of the athlete's drugs test?' and quite rightly so in my opinion. Well, back then things were

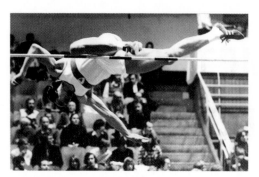

Fig 1.1 An athlete performing the straddle jump technique.

different and on this occasion a new shoe design was at the centre of the world's athletics media attention. The accusation, by the Americans, was that the Soviets were using a built up sole that gave Stepanov a mechanical advantage at take-off. The Americans claimed this shoe was the reason for the Soviet athlete's new record, and thus it should still be held by the USA. The International Amateur Athletic Federation (IAAF) was forced to step in and implement a new rule to restrict the sole height of all future high jump shoes to 13mm. However, the record still stood, much to the dismay of the Americans.

As you would expect, normal order resumed in 1960 and American athlete John Thomas reclaimed the world record, pushing it to 2.23m and making him the overwhelming favourite for the Rome Olympics to be held later that year. Dyachkov, however, had other ideas.

Yuri Verkhoshansky was a young, relatively unknown coach who had a lot of respect for Dyachkov. Towards the end of the 1950s, Verkhoshanksy was training a group of student track and field athletes from the Aeronautical Engineering Institute in Moscow. The institute had no indoor athletic training facilities and, faced with the harsh Russian winters, Verkhoshanksy decided to train his athletes in the warmer corridors and stairwells of the institute's building. This lack of space led to the athletes being split into two groups, with one performing jumping exercises in the corridors and the other barbell exercises in the stairwell. The most frequently used strength exercise was the barbell squat and the most frequently used jump exercise was a short run-up with a double leg take-off, where the athlete's aim was to touch the ceiling. At first, his athletes could only just reach with their fingertips but, after a short period of training, Verkhoshansky's athletes were able to get their palm flat on the ceiling. During this period, Verkhoshansky was taking a particular interest in the triple jump and the biomechanics and loading during the hop, step and jump phases. He discovered that the enormous pressure or downward force experienced by triple jumpers on the last contact phase was upwards of 300kg. This led him to think about how he could replicate this force so he could train his athletes to overcome it and therefore improve their overall jump performance. Verkhoshansky experimented with many different barbell exercises as he looked for an exercise to replicate this force that all his athletes could perform.

The first exercise he tried was a simple barbell half squat. However, this led to his taller athletes complaining of lower back pain at the excessive weights that Verkhoshansky was trying to get them to replicate. He then experimented with variations of the leg press but not on a leg press machine that you would find in a performance gym today. Athletes would lay on their back with their feet in the air and, with some help, they would balance the barbell across the soles of their feet while trying to press the bar vertically. Even with two assistants at the sides, this exercise was deemed too dangerous (surprise, surprise!) for fear of it falling on to the athlete below and crushing them.

It was at this point, with his limited 'corridor' training facilities and basic equipment, that Verkhoshansky had his eureka moment and developed what is probably the single most important exercise for any athlete wanting to attain speed and power – the depth jump. This very high intensity exercise uses the kinetic energy of the falling athlete to increase the downward force upon landing. This allowed Verkhoshansky to replicate the huge forces experienced by his athletes during jumping and thus train specifically for improved jump height. This method of training was called 'the shock method'.

Dyachkov rarely published his training methods during his early coaching years but his decades of studying high jump technique had led him to use similar barbell exercise methods to Verkhoshansky. Dyachkov's advice has been credited as a major influence on the infamous 1961 paper by Verkhoshansky, 'The barbell in the training of track field jumpers'. In 1962, Dyachkov finally published his paper where he presented his 'conjugated method' of training. This involved using barbell exercises in athletes' training to improve the technical skill of high jumpers. This article caught the eye of Verkhoshansky who, ever the forward-thinking coach, set out to explore Dyachkov's ideas further with the aim of formulating the criteria for selecting the weight exercises.

Both coaches respected each other greatly, however the reality was that Dyachkov was head coach of the Soviet national team and Verkhoshansky was now coach of the Student Moscow Team. The resources available to the respective coaches were very different, with Dyachkov having all the benefits of indoor training facilities and Verkhoshansky just that of a corridor and a stairwell. Barbell exercises were therefore used very differently. Dyachkov used them as part of the athletes' technical preparation, whereas Verkhoshansky had to spend entire sessions just performing weight training and jumps due to his limited resources. The Verkhoshanksy method of using barbell and jumping exercises in the same training session were instrumental in developing athletes with 'muscles of a deer rather than those of a buffalo', as he used to phrase it. Previous thinking had led coaches to believe that increased muscle mass would slow an athlete down due to him becoming big and bulky like a bodybuilder – the traditional purpose of lifting weights. Verkhoshansky's methods proved this to be untrue. His new methods of training such as the vertical drop-rebound jump, or depth jump as it is now known, led to a huge increase in the level of performance in his athletes' track and field events. Working as the head coach of the Moscow United Team, Verkhoshansky's athlete Bros Zubov became the European and Soviet record holder in the sprint events and led to Verkhoshansky being appointed as the 'Honoured Coach of Russia'.

Are you still wondering about the result of the 1960s Rome Olympics high jump competition I mentioned earlier? Well, having read this introduction I am sure you will not be surprised when I tell you it was not won by John Thomas of the USA. He came third behind, yes you've guessed it, two Soviet athletes. Robert Shavlakadze and Valeri Brumel, who took gold and silver and, yes you've guessed it again, they were coached by none other than Dyachkov. By 1963, the Russian athlete Brumel had raised the world record to 2.28m, still only competing on a dirt track and landing on a sawdust pit. Brumel's superior strength and speed was thanks to his training and the methods developed by both Dyachkov and Verkhoshansky. There was no sign of any built-up shoe for anyone to complain about or any controversy whatsoever, just superior training techniques that got results.

The word plyometrics is from the literal translation from the Greek meaning to increase measure (*plio* – more; *plythein* – increase; *metric* – measure). It was first used in 1975 by Fred Wilt of the United States while observing Soviet athletes warming up. Wilt, a respected runner and coach, wanted to know more about this new training concept helping the Soviets to dominate not just track and field but gymnastics and weightlifting in the 1970s. Wilt reached out to fellow coach and scholar Dr Michael Yessis. Dr Yessis had previously introduced the concept of shock training to the United States through the study and translation of none other than the 'Godfather of plyometrics', as he now considered Verkhoshansky. In 1982, Yessis had travelled to the Soviet Union to work with Verkhoshansky and learn his methods of developing speed and power. Wilt's and Yessis's keen interest in plyometrics inspired their collaboration to educate and ensure this information was available to US coaches to help them improve the performance of the nation's athletes. Their publication *Soviet Theory, Technique and Training for Running and Hurdling* was published in 1984 and, as such, Wilt and Dr Yessis can truly be regarded as the West's pioneers of plyometrics training.

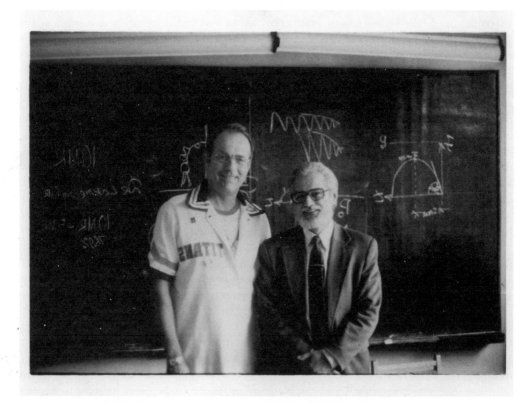

Fig 1.2 Fred Wilt and Dr Michael Yessis, the pioneers of Western plyometrics training.
(Printed with kind permission of Dr Michael Yessis)

2 | THE SCIENCE BEHIND PLYOMETRICS

All coaches and athletes are looking to run faster, jump higher, kick or hit further, throw or punch harder. Once your technique is perfected, these individual performance objectives are more often than not determined by the holy grail of training – more power. Unfortunately these days many athletes focus too much of their training programmes on lifting heavy weights. I am not saying these gym-based exercises are incorrect or indeed bad for you as an athlete, as they do have their place in improving power performance through muscular and nervous system adaptations. However, they are not really the most efficient way of developing power directly. Before we start to look at how to train specifically for improved power, we should first take a moment to understand what it is.

THE THEORY OF ATHLETIC POWER

Power is the combination of strength and speed and there are two types of power that relate to sports performance – maximal power and power endurance. From a training viewpoint, these are two very different objectives when designing a training programme. Maximal power is 'the ability to exert a maximal force in as short a time as possible', whereas power endurance is 'the rate at which force is applied over a period of time with a minimal reduction in quality of effort'. If you take a look at Table 1, you will see almost all sports involve either maximal power or power endurance.

Power is considered to be the measured rate of performing work, with 'work' in relation to sports and exercise simply referring to the specific exercise or movement such as jumping, kicking, punching and so on. In order to measure the energy cost of this work, power measures the size of the force applied and the velocity at which it is applied for each second that 'work' is being performed.

To understand the power equation from a training perspective we need to look at what 'work' is in relation to performance. Work [W] is defined scientifically as the 'application of force over some distance'. In simple terms it's the action of performing the required task – work. So, and this is fairly obvious, the faster you run a known distance, the further you throw an implement such as a javelin or the harder you punch or even block an opponent, the more power you will have exerted.

Let's rewrite the power equation to be more

MAXIMAL POWER	POWER ENDURANCE
The ability to exert a maximal force in as short a time as possible. Single efforts of specific movement patterns. Accelerating, jumping and throwing implements.	The rate at which force is applied over a period of time with a minimal reduction in quality of effort Repeated efforts of specific movement patterns. Sprinting, hitting (racket sports), repeated punching.

Table 1   The two types of athletic power.

The Power Equation

$$\text{Power [P]} = \frac{\text{Work [W]}}{\text{Time [T]}}$$

Fig 2.2 The power equation.

The Athletic Training Power Equation

$$\frac{\text{Force [F] x Distance [D]}}{\text{Time [T]}}$$

Fig 2.3 The athletic training power equation.

training specific and examine each of its constituent parts.

0. **Force (F)** is the capacity to move an object with a known mass. This can be a person's weight when referring to bodyweight movements such as sprinting, jumping or bounding exercises or the total weight of an object that is being moved such as a barbell, medicine ball or throwing implement such

12

as a javelin. Force is measured in Newtons. [1kg = 10 Newtons]

1. **Distance (D)** is how far a person or object travels. This is the recorded maximal distance effort of, for example, a vertical or horizontal jump or throw. Distance is measured in metres.
2. **The time (T)** it takes to move the Force [F] the recorded distance [D]. Time is measured in seconds.

This equation simply means that to increase power an athlete will have to increase the speed at which this force is applied over the required distance. Just increasing the ability to apply force through strength alone will not result in more power. For instance, when looking to increase force all coaches and athletes will turn to traditional weight room exercises such as maximal strength, low repetition heavy squats, step-ups or bench. Now remember the first paragraph of this chapter: 'Unfortunately these days many athletes spend too much of their athletic training programmes focused on lifting heavy weights.' The reason for this statement is that these exercises do not allow the athlete to move at speed. A traditional weight exercise has an initial acceleration phase, where maximum force is applied as the movement is initiated, followed by a deceleration as the weight passes through the sticking point and a final deceleration as the weight is stopped by the athlete at the end range of motion. This need to slow the weight at the end of range is to ensure the exercise is performed correctly, with control also helping to limit the chances of injury. Although this is, of course, correct and extremely necessary, this type of exercise limits the ability to apply speed to a movement and therefore reduces the ability to apply and train for true power.

If increasing strength alone is not the route to the holy grail of power, let's concentrate on increasing our speed of movement in training. Surely that will give us more power – or will it? Just concentrating on the speed of a movement alone will not increase your power output. This may sound confusing but it's quite simple. Take a look at the force-velocity curve below and it will all start to click into place.

Still confused? Look at the graph again and notice the two measured variables on the axis – force and velocity. Remember that force *is the capacity to move an object with a known mass* and velocity *is the rate of change of the positioning of an object, taking into account its speed and direction of motion.* Let's relate this to an athletic movement such as a counter movement jump. The more force and velocity I apply when I jump, the more power I will achieve and the higher I will jump. If I apply more force than velocity or more velocity than force my jump will not be as powerful and subsequently not as high.

Improved Power

Shifting the force-velocity curve to the right ultimately means you are applying greater force at higher velocities. This shift will result in an athlete being able to run faster, jump higher or throw further.

Understanding the relationship between force and velocity is paramount to improving power. As you can see from the force-velocity curve, the more force you apply the less velocity is realized and, inversely, the more velocity you apply the less force is applied. Power sits in the middle, which basically means equal measures of force and velocity must be achieved to realize optimum power. Therefore, the goal of any coach or athlete wishing to improve power must be to shift the force-velocity curve to the right, increasing equal but improved measures of both. In other words, to increase power you must apply greater force at higher velocities.

Plyometric exercises do not limit force or velocity due to the nature of the exercises. Jumps and throws require no deceleration at the end of the movement. Think of it like an

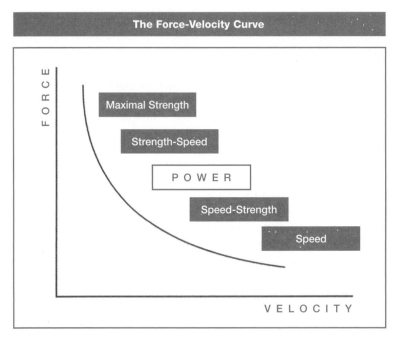

Fig 2.4 The force-velocity curve.

elastic band – you pre-stretch an elastic band to ping it across a room and that's exactly what you do with plyometric training. Using this theory and understanding it is, of course, possible to make an exercise such as a bench press plyometric. Lower the barbell to your chest and then press it upwards as quickly as possible, letting go of the bar at the end of range when the hands are furthest away from the chest. This letting go or chest throw of the bar ensures there is no slowing down of the movement, making it truly explosive and fundamentally plyometric. There are, however, practical problems and safety issues involved. You will, of course, need a trusted training partner to catch the upward moving bar before gravity takes effect and the bar makes its way back towards your head! If you can't think of anyone to perform this task or you are indeed attached to your head and would like to remain so, then you could of course perform a plyometric press-up as it's the same in principle, or is it?

Let's think about a plyometric push-up with regards to the force-velocity curve and in what circumstance that last statement is untrue. The fundamental question you need to ask yourself is: what is the readiness for the athlete to train? For example, in the instance that an athlete does not have enough strength to perform a body weight push-up or multiple reps easily with control then straightaway it could be said the athlete will not be able to apply enough force. In addition to this, how would they be able to apply enough speed to the press-up to increase its velocity and achieve optimum power? The simple answer, of course, is they can't. From a coaching perspective, anyone who cannot perform a body weight push-up with control should not be performing a plyometric push-up. Unfortunately these days you will often see coaches dishing out plyo push-ups for punishment during an unsuccessful tactical or technical session on the pitch or sometimes as part of a high intensity interval training circuit session with athletes who do not have the required base strength. In my opinion, all athletes should be able to perform the body weight equivalent of that movement for at least twenty reps before starting out on a plyometric variation of the same exercise. You can read more about this in Chapter 4.

THE PHYSIOLOGY OF POWER

Most coaches and athletes understand what power is but unfortunately many fail to understand the simple muscle physiology behind it.

We won't spend time talking about what muscles are made up of as I really want to ensure that as a coach or athlete you get to grips with how muscles work with regards to plyometrics. There are plenty of good physiology books and websites out there that will tell you everything you need to know and in more depth than what we would cover in a few paragraphs. So let's get back to practical plyometric understanding.

There are three types of muscle contractions that you must be aware of for plyometric training: concentric, eccentric and isometric.

- **Concentric Muscle Contraction** – A type of muscle activation that increases tension on a muscle as it shortens. Concentric contractions are the most common types of muscle activation athletes perform in a gym when they lift weights.
- **Eccentric Muscle Contraction** – A type of muscle activation that increases tension on a muscle as it lengthens. Eccentric contractions typically occur when a muscle opposes a stronger force, which causes the muscle to lengthen as it contracts such as lowering yourself during a pull-up exercise.
- **Isometric Muscle Contraction** – A type of muscle activation in which the muscle fires but there is no movement at a joint. In this type of muscle contraction, there is no change in length of the muscle, and no movement at the joints. An example of

isometric exercise includes pushing against a wall or a plank exercise.

Remember these types of contractions as you will need this knowledge in a minute. Now, let's think about a counter movement jump for a moment. What movement occurs when you jump, which joints are involved, how do your muscles work and what actions are involved?

It is generally agreed in the science community that all plyometric sequences follow the same process of a pre-stretch or loading followed by rapid muscle contraction or unloading. This process is also known as the stretch-shortening cycle. However, understanding plyometrics just through the physical limb movements that take place is where most coaches and athletes go wrong in their understanding of plyometrics. This definition of plyometrics would lead us to believe that a counter movement jump is a two phase process – bending simultaneously at the hips, knees and ankles (loading) then powerfully straightening your legs to get maximum upward momentum to leave the ground (unloading) – and you'd be right, but only when it comes to actual limb movement. As a coach or athlete, your primary objective in training is to induce physiological adaptions to muscles or energy systems in order to improve performance. Think again about the muscle actions we talked about earlier. Which ones occur during jumping? That's right, all of them.

When you look at explosive movements such as a counter movement jump the stretch-shortening cycle actually has three phases and is sometimes referred to as being triphasic. Some authors have described plyometric movements as a five-phase process with a 'momentum phase' at either end of the triphasic description. This is not incorrect, and in my opinion a more accurate description of what is actually taking place with regards to technique, but for the purpose of this book we will stick to triphasic in order to focus on the actual plyometric muscle actions taking place.

THE STRETCH-SHORTENING CYCLE		
Eccentric Phase	Transition Phase	Concentric Phase
Amortization Phase		
Loading Phase	Coupling Phase	Unloading Phase
Muscle Action		
Eccentric	Isometric	Concentric
The muscles lengthens or stretches – stores elastic energy and stimulates the muscles spindles	No muscle movement occurs – the time that elapses before the concentric phase starts – Signals are sent to the spinal cord from muscles spindles and musculoskeletal organs (GTO) and back for more dynamic muscle contractions	The muscle contracts, rapidly utilizing the stored elastic energy

Table 2   The plyometric sequence.

Still thinking 'why is it triphasic?' Well, take a look at Table 2. As you can see, the action of a counter movement jump requires a loading phase where the muscles lengthen eccentrically, in this case the gluteals, quadriceps and calves. There is also a coupling phase, where no movement occurs and when the isometric muscle action takes place, and an unloading phase, in which the muscles contract rapidly to achieve upward movement.

LOADING PHASE

The first phase of a plyometric movement involves actions that eccentrically load the working muscle. The stretched muscle stores elastic energy due to the load applied to the joint. Without this pre-stretch of the muscle no energy can be stored in the muscle and subsequently no plyometric activity can occur. The loading phase is finished when the eccentric movement reaches its end. In the example of the counter movement jump, this would be when the athlete reaches the bottom part of the movement.

COUPLING PHASE

During the second phase no movement takes place. This is an extremely short part of the plyometric sequence and is the point at which movement changes from eccentric muscle contractions to concentric muscle contractions or from the loading to the unloading phase. Also known as the transmission phase, this rapid phase must join together the loading and unloading phase seamlessly, ensuring stored elastic energy is not lost through heat due to a slow change in direction of the movement. You cannot see this phase with the naked eye, for our counter movement jump sequence the optimum time for the coupling phase is between 15 to 23 milliseconds to ensure a powerful and quick transmission to the unloading phase.

UNLOADING PHASE

Once the loading and coupling phases have taken place, the unloading phase is executed caused by the concentric muscle actions and subsequent shortening of the muscle-tendon unit. It is the total effect of the three physiological muscle mechanisms that is responsible for optimal power generation during the unloading phase.

MUSCLE MECHANISMS RESPONSIBLE FOR PLYOMETRIC POWER

During the stretch-shortening cycle there are three physiological muscle mechanisms at the loading phase that help to increase force output.

Muscle Potentiation

This is standard muscle physiology. As the muscle lengthens the muscles contractile properties increase due to the sarcomere becoming stretched. This increases cross bridge formation as the thin (actin) filament and the thick (myosin) filament move closer together. These actin and myosin filaments are also known as the series elastic components (SEC).

Stretch Reflex

When muscles are stretched the muscles' spindles and musculoskeletal organs such as the Golgi tendon organ (GTO), a sensory receptor that lies in the tendon, send a signal to the spinal cord, which then returns inhibitory feedback to the muscle for more dynamic contractions.

Stored Elastic Energy

Elastic energy, sometimes referred to as mechanical energy, is stored in the series elastic components of the muscle during the eccentric phase of a movement. This energy is then released during the concentric phase. The tendon of a muscle, however, has been shown to be the main contributor to the changes in length of a muscle-tendon unit and the storage of elastic potential energy. A muscle's elasticity and healthy tendons are therefore extremely important to plyometric ability. A muscle-tendon unit that is able to lengthen and increase in tension and readily return to its original state with greater force, efficiency or both is more beneficial for athletic power. Every athlete must therefore ensure they not only have strong muscles but also flexible and supple muscles if they wish to increase plyometric performance.

Something to think about!

Interestingly it has been found that, where a muscle crosses one joint (mono-articular) such as the soleus with the ankle, it has been shown to elicit more stretch reflex than that of the gastrocnemius muscle that crosses two joints (biarticular) – the ankle and knee. For instance, in our counter movement jump example you will get more *stretch* across the soleus muscle than you would in a gastocnemius muscle by the simple fact the knee is bent and therefore not providing maximal stretch to the whole muscle. This in turn reduces muscle potentiation, the stretch reflex and, of course, its stored elastic energy. So you should always think about which muscles are involved in athletic movement, how many joints they cross, the actions of the muscles and whether they are truly plyometric.

THINGS TO REMEMBER...

- You must have equal measure of velocity and force to ensure optimal power.
- Plyometric exercises do not limit force or velocity due to the nature of the exercises.
- All plyometric movements are triphasic and include a loading, coupling and unloading phase.
- Plyometric exercise uses three muscle contractions – eccentric, isometric and concentric.
- The three muscle mechanisms responsible for plyometric performance are: muscle potentiation, stretch reflex and stored elastic energy.

3 | WHAT ARE PLYOMETRICS?

Plyometrics are exercises that require muscles to exert maximum force in as short a time as possible with the goal of increasing both speed and power. True plyometrics engage the nervous system with the stretch reflex and plyometric effect occurring predominately in the muscle tendon rather than the muscle itself. Plyometric exercises should be performed for between one (single response drills) and ten reps (multiple response drills). The very nature of the words 'explosive force' would lead anyone to understand the reasons behind this as you cannot maintain maximal or near maximal power over long periods of time. It is also recommended that any plyometric exercise or drill lasts for no more than ten seconds. This 'timed' guideline is linked to the energy systems used in exercise and, as we all know, it is the creatine phosphate system that is utilized in explosive events lasting for ten seconds or less.

LOWER BODY PLYOMETRICS

There are six different types of lower body plyometric exercises that increase in intensity due to the nature and forces involved. There are exceptions to the rules but they start with jumps in place and continue with standing jumps, multiple hops and jumps, bounding, box drills and, finally, depth jumps.

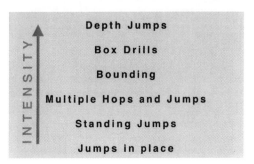

Fig 3.1 Types of lower body plyometric exercise.

JUMPS IN PLACE

As the name suggests, you jump and land in the same place. These jumps are relatively low in intensity and are a great starting place for teaching correct jumping and landing mechanics while building the athlete's confidence. There are some great footwork drills, also considered to be 'jumps in place', that can be practised by the athlete to increase their reactivity and gain good balance and proprioception before moving on to more complex and demanding drills.

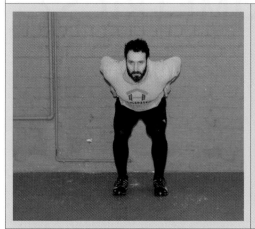 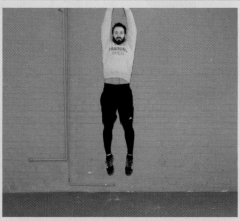

The athlete jumps in a vertical direction landing in the same spot and position as they started in.

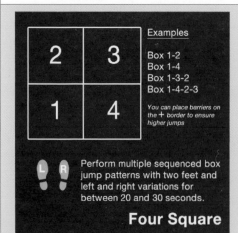 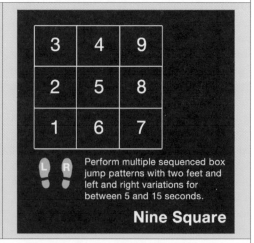

Footwork drills lasting no more than ten seconds can be used to develop an athlete's plyometric competency. These are considered to be jumps in place due to the fact there is no linear travel.

Low Intensity

Table 3 Plyometric exercises.

STANDING JUMPS
These single efforts can be in any direction and are focused on developing lower body power. A maximal effort jump that focuses on correct technique and speed of movement.

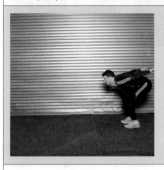 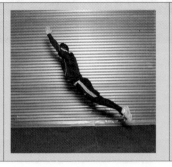 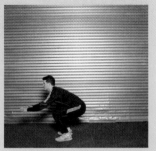

The athlete jumps in a vertical or horizontal direction and is focused on single maximum effort, in other words how high or far can you jump.
Low to Medium Intensity

MULTIPLE HOPS AND JUMPS
A progression from jumps in place and standing jumps, these multiple response drills require total control and emphasis on good technique to benefit the athlete.

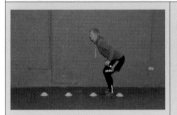 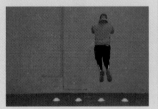 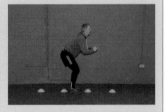

The athlete jumps with repeated efforts in a vertical or horizontal direction They should be performed over distances between 10 to 30m.
Medium Intensity

Table 3 *Continued.*

BOUNDING

Often seen as 'triple jump' training, this multiple response drill will help to develop lower body power for increased speed and acceleration.

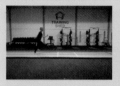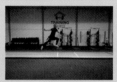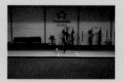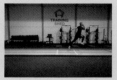

Typically used by runners or any bipedal sports, bounding exercises stress a specific aspect of the running cycle. They usually occur over distances greater than 30m and look to improve stride length and frequency.

Medium Intensity

BOX DRILLS

These exercises and drills are, of course, plyometric when performed at the correct intensity and rest periods. More often than not, it is these drills that become a jump training or conditioning drills. Misguided athletes will often complete multiple jumps for more than the recommend ten seconds, often for minutes on end. There is nothing wrong with this if your objective is to increase fitness and conditioning but for plyometrics they must be focused on explosiveness, rather than in ninety second-plus fitness drills!

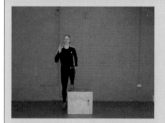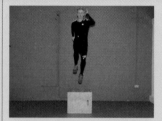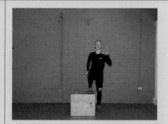

Box drills combine multiple hops and jumps with depth jumps. They can be both vertical and horizontal.

Low to High Intensity (dependent on box height)

DEPTH JUMPS

The holy grail of plyometrics! This exercise uses an athlete's body weight, gravity and ground reaction forces to develop power. Depth jumps are very high intensity and you should therefore ensure you have the correct height box for each athlete. It is also important to have performed numerous plyometric sessions to build up the correct strength and technique before attempting this highly demanding exercise.

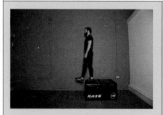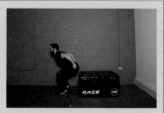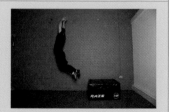

Depth jumps use an athlete's body weight and gravity to exert force against the ground.

High Intensity

Table 3 *Continued.*

These are just exercises on their own but when linked to movement patterns in sport they become essential tools in the development of specific speed and power. So let's look at movement patterns that occur in sport requiring speed and power.

- **Starting Speed** – the ability of an athlete to go from a stopped or non-moving state to a moving or mobile state. This is sometimes referred to by coaches and sports scientists as first step quickness and usually refers to the first 5m. Gaining an advantage over your opponent in this movement skill is often all you need, such as being first to the ball or leaving your race opponent standing.
- **Acceleration** – the ability of an athlete to reach maximal speed, under control, in the shortest amount of time. There are two ways to improve acceleration: increasing an athlete's stride length and/or stride frequency. Stride length is the amount of distance covered by one full stride of an athlete, and stride frequency is how fast an athlete can turn over the limb to produce another stride. Plyometrics will improve both of these.
- **Change of Direction** – sometimes referred to as agility, it is the ability to move and change the position of the body quickly and effectively while under control.
- **Vertical Jump** – is the act of raising your centre of gravity higher in the vertical plane through jumping.
- **Horizontal Jump** – the act of jumping and propelling the body to land in a forward position, such as in the long jump or performing a diving header or catch.

Now we have identified some athletic movement skills essential to sports performance you should consider which ones take place during your chosen sport. Ask yourself the following questions. Does my sport require good starting speed or acceleration? How about changes in direction? Is there any vertical or horizontal jumping involved? Take some time to do a simple needs analysis of your sport. There is no need to break movement down with sports science or biomechanics focused

	Starting Speed	Acceleration	Changes in direction	Vertical Jumping	Horizontal Jumping
Sprinting with the ball in a straight line as fast as possible from a static position	X	X			
Accelerating in a straight line with the ball while running		X			
Accelerating in a straight line to close down an opponent with/without the ball starting from a static position	X	X			
Chasing an opponent down from a static position to make a tackle/intercept a pass	X	X	X		
Chasing an opponent down from an already moving position to make a tackle/intercept a pass		X	X		
Challenging for an attacking or defensive header				X	X

Table 4 **Example of actions that occur for outfield players in football.**

terminology – just narrate all the movements that occur in your sport and then tick which of the athletic skills we have identified are involved.

This process is simple when it comes to sports such as track and field and given the history of the development of plyometrics (see Chapter 1) you can understand why these sports' coaches and athletes use plyometric training as an essential tool for improving performance. A sprinter will require starting speed and acceleration. A high jumper will require vertical jumping and a long jumper horizontal jumping. That's all pretty obvious and self-explanatory but what about team sports?

A quick overview of the world's most popular game, football (see Table 4), shows that of all the athletic skills previously mentioned, a footballer would benefit from developing not just one, as in some of the athletics events, but every movement skill previously identified.

CONNECTING PLYOMETRIC EXERCISES TO IMPROVING ATHLETIC MOVEMENT SKILLS

We have identified that sports require the development of more powerful athletic movement skills in order to compete but which plyometric exercises should you use in train-ing to help improve them? Table 5 is probably the single most important table for planning your plyometric training. This links together which plyometric exercises you should be using to improve your identified athletic movement skills, ensuring you select the right exercises and drills.

UPPER BODY PLYOMETRICS

Although plyometrics are generally regarded as lower body exercises by many coaches and athletes, it is the action of the muscle, a loading and coupling followed by a rapid unload, which makes an exercise plyometric. Therefore there is no reason why the upper body cannot be trained in the same way.

Upper body plyometrics are grouped into push exercises and medicine ball exercises. The advantage of the medicine ball exercises are that you can control the intensity through the load using medicine balls of different weight. These exercises are more dynamic than the single plane of movement push-up exercises and can include trunk training through the use of rotational medicine ball drills, which helps to develop a strong core and greater power transfer throughout the body. The plyometric push exercises are generally restricted to body weight loading or involve single arm movements and are therefore regarded as high intensity.

SKILL	Plyometric Exercise						
	Jumps in Place	Standing Jumps	Multiple Jumps	Bounding	Box Drills	Bounding	Depth Jumps
Starting Speed	✓	✓	✓				✓
Acceleration			✓	✓	✓	✓	
Change of Direction		✓	✓		✓		✓
Vertical Jump	✓	✓	✓		✓		✓
Horizontal Jump		✓	✓	✓	✓	✓	

Table 5   Which plyometric exercises build which athletic movement skills?

MEDICINE BALL EXERCISES
Remember the requirements of a plyometric exercise before designing multiple rep plyometric med ball exercises. Plyometric med ball exercises can include throws, slams, drops and passes.
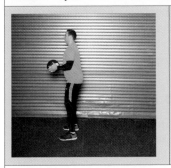 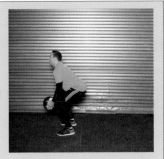 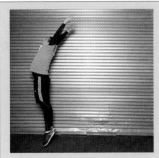
Medicine ball exercises can include horizontal, vertical, diagonal, arced and twisting movement patterns. They can also be combined with lower body plyometrics.
Low to High Intensity (Dependent on Load)

PUSH EXERCISES
The use of weight bags or body weight through press-ups is a good way to develop upper body plyometric power.
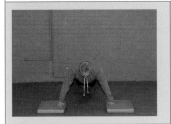 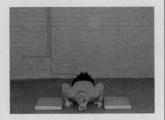 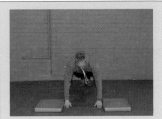
These can include traditional push-ups, shoulder presses and drop push-up movement patterns, as well as single arm exercises.
High Intensity

Table 6   Upper body plyometric exercises.

Most sports require some form of upper body plyometric training. Those that require the use of push exercises include martial arts, javelin, shot put, boxing, rugby and American football. Trunk training is essential in all these sports as well as sports such as canoeing, kayaking, any bipedal sport that requires efficient power transfer during running and sprinting, swimming and even cycling. The body's core is the foundation for all movement and stabilizes the thoracic cage and pelvis during dynamic athletic movements. An efficient core provides good strength, stability and mobility, ensuring optimal efficiency of the entire kinetic chain during movements and giving dynamic stabilization to acceleration and deceleration. It

25

is also the foundation of proximal stability to movements of the extremities such as throwing and kicking. In essence, if you are not currently using medicine ball exercises in your training plans then you should start today.

SINGLE RESPONSE DRILLS

When starting out with plyometric drills, single response drills are always the place to start. Being able to perform a perfect technique for these types of exercises and drills is a great platform for developing your plyometric skills before embarking on more complex drills. Remember: always get the basics right before you progress on to more complex drills. You learned to walk before you could run so make sure you can execute a simple single response drill such as hopping on the spot before you start hopping down a track. Single response drills are maximal effort exercises with the aim of achieving maximal power. There are rest periods between each effort, with each drill performed in short sets to maintain power and avoid muscle fatigue.

MULTIPLE RESPONSE DRILLS

These more complex drills involve multiple efforts of the same movement. They can be performed over distance or repeated vertically for lower body plyometrics. They can also be repeated throws to a partner or solid surface when performing upper body plyo-

metrics. Multiple response drills can include both single and double leg jumps, often with changes of direction to replicate sports specific movements. Equipment such as hurdles and boxes is commonly used to provide external stimulus and make exercises more demanding of the athlete. Simple bounds and hops are also multiple response drills.

THINGS TO REMEMBER

The following athletic skills can be improved by plyometric training:

- Starting speed
- Acceleration
- Changes in direction
- Vertical jumping
- Horizontal jumping.

Lower body plyometrics include jumps in place, standing jumps, multiple hops and jump, bounding, box drills and, finally, depth jumps.

Upper body plyometrics include push exercises and medicine ball exercises.

Most sports require medicine ball or trunk training exercises to increase power transfer during athletic movements and will increase the efficiency of both lower and upper body plyometrics.

Always start with single response drills before progressing to multiple response drills.

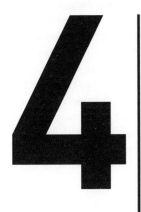

BEFORE YOU BEGIN

Plyometrics are probably one of the most misunderstood and misused training modalities in developing athletic performance. They are often referred to as being dangerous and responsible for muscle strains when actually it is the coaches' and athletes' understanding that is at fault. All too often, negative opinions are formed due to bad experiences. Unfortunately this is often linked to an excessive volume of work, incorrect selection of plyometric drills for the athletes' needs and the physical unpreparedness of the athlete for this type of training.

Before you embark on a plyometric training programme, there are some guidelines I believe you should follow. In order to better understand the correct application of plyometrics, the National Strength and Conditioning Association's position statement is a good place to start. There is, of course, every chance that even at low intensities joints can be exposed to potential injury if the athlete does not possess sufficient muscular strength and neuromuscular control. There are many thoughts as to what level of strength an athlete should possess, ranging from a simple body weight squat to a back squat at 1½ to 2½ times body weight and even a rapid squat at 60 per cent body weight for five reps in five seconds.

Unfortunately, many opinions on what this level should be are simply that – opinions. Research is still limited with most of the current advice available only applicable to male athletes in their prime. This fails to address masters athletes, women and, worst of all, children. Training that is specific or similar to the activity being performed is believed to be optimal. When you compete in a sport that includes movements that elicit plyometric properties such as jumping and sprinting with ground reaction forces up to seven times a person's body mass surely this should warrant some form of plyometric training?

PHYSICAL LIMITATIONS

Plyometrics require total body control. If you have suffered previous injuries to any of the joints involved in plyometric exercises then this could limit your training capacity. Flexibility is key to the muscle's ability to utilize the forces experienced during the loading and rapid unloading during fast movement patterns such as plyometrics. Joint stability, balance and proprioception are all vital components of athletic training and any restrictions in these areas could impair your progress.

A simple postural assessment could identify areas that need to be addressed through strength training to ensure a solid initial platform for developing athletic ability. It is never good to judge a person's athletic training readiness on their age. Some athletes may have achieved success on natural talent or hereditary genetic advantages alone and using their age to determine their readiness to train is both incorrect and potentially dangerous. In general fitness terms, you should be able to exercise for several minutes continuously with anthropo-metrics typical of an athletic body. Overweight athletes may cause excessive impacts to their joints, especially during landing mechanics for lower body plyometrics. Being able to control your own body weight and in all planes of movement is often considered a prerequisite of athletic training. In addition to this, coaches and athletes must remember there are obvious differences between men and women owing to their genetic make-up. The length of a limb or the percentage of fast twitch muscle fibres are all dictated by genetics, so everyone has a

National Strength and Conditioning Association

Plyometric Position Statement

1. The stretch-shortening cycle, characterized by rapid deceleration of a mass followed almost immediately by rapid acceleration of mass in the opposite direction is essential in the performance of most competitive sports, particularly those involving running, jumping and rapid changes in direction

2. A plyometric exercise programme – which trains the muscles, connective tissue and nervous system to carry out effectively the stretch-shortening cycle – can improve performance in most competitive sports

3. A plyometric training programme for athletes should include sport-specific exercises

4. Carefully applied plyometric exercise programmes are no more harmful than other forms of sport training and competition and may be necessary for safe adaptation to the rigours of 'explosive' sports

5. Only athletes who have already achieved high levels of strength through standard resistance training should engage in plyometric drills

6. Depth jumps should only be used by a small percentage of athletes engaged in plyometric training. As a rule, athletes weighing more than 220lb should not depth jump from platforms higher than 18in

7. Plyometric drills affecting a particular muscle/joint complex should not be performed on consecutive days

8. Plyometric drills should not be performed when an athlete is fatigued. Time for complete recovery should be allowed between plyometric exercise sets

9. Footwear and landing surfaces used in plyometric drills must have good shock absorbing qualities

10. A thorough set of warm-up exercises should be performed before beginning a plyometric training session. Less demanding drills should be mastered prior to attempting more complex and intense drills

Explosive/Plyometric Exercises. National Strength and Conditioning Association

limit. Some companies such as DNAFit are now offering non-invasive DNA tests that will give you a report detailing your genetic make-up. Maybe this is the future of applied training, although it will take many years to justify this through scientific research.

CHILDREN AND PLYOMETRICS

Often believed to be a no-go area in training, academic scholars now believe coaching plyometrics may actually be a good thing. The development of sound motor skills are more readily absorbed by children during their 'skill-hungry' years. Their neuromuscular system is developing fast and learning coordinated movements can enhance this development as well as stand them in good stead for future training programmes. As a child, I am sure many of you have performed a star jump or played hopscotch and my simple question is: why as coaches should we be anti-explosive for youth athletic programmes – are these simple games not plyometric? I would always advocate that correct movement skills and of course appropriate loading are the key to any training programme, whatever your age.

With this is mind, I would recommend simple beginner plyometric drills start with two feet drills and any loading be no more than 1 to 2kg in the case of medicine ball training. As the child develops physically and technically, it is possible to move to single leg and higher intensity drills but only if they are ready and show correct technique. A progressive training programme from simple to complex training drills should be observed. As a child transitions through puberty it is often observed that he or she starts to elicit incorrect techniques and can appear clumsy and uncoordinated. At this stage of development it can be good to reinforce movement skills but it is advised that caution prevails as during high periods of growth, also known as peak height velocity or PHV, it is possible a child can become both uncoordinated and frustrated while also having

There are many myths surrounding the prescription of plyometrics with youth athletes. Here are three of my favourites:

Myth 1

Plyometric training is unsafe and dangerous for children.

Fact: As long as a plyometric programme is designed by a qualified professional taking into consideration the athlete's ability and specificity there is no greater risk of injury than any other form of training. Performing simple jumps in place and progressing safely and appropriately will ensure a well-rounded programme of athletic development.

Myth 2

Children who have not reached puberty should not perform plyometrics

Fact: Children can start plyometric training when they are considered to have the emotional maturity to accept and follow directions.

Myth 3

Plyometrics will cause bone growth plate damage

Fact: There is not one single report of growth plate damage during resistance training studies that have been designed and delivered by a qualified and knowledgeable coach. Younger children are also said to be more resilient to shearing (unaligned) type forces such as jumping and bounding.

a higher propensity to injury due to their reduced level of control and proprioception.

As with any plyometrics programme, complete rest should be observed between exercises and drills, allowing for total recovery. It is advisable to start with repetitions of between six and ten and complete only one to two sets depending on the current athletic ability of the child. Plyometrics should never be over prescribed and there should be at the very least one day's complete rest between sessions. I would normally err on the side of caution and enforce two to three days of non-plyometric activity, especially for young beginners. Plyometrics is a form of resistance training and must therefore follow the typical principles of progressive overload – the systematic increase in training frequency, volume and intensity. With the correct supervision and instruction the use of plyometrics by children is both safe, fun and essential in developing true athletic potential. How many of today's champion athletes, although they may not have known they were doing 'plyometrics' when they were children, started with these types of drills. At my best guess I would say most of them.

MASTERS ATHLETES

A decline in athletic ability is inevitable as one gets older and as such plyometric programmes should include no more than five low-to-moderate intensity exercises. The volume of exercises should also be lower and the total contacts in a session reduced compared to that of a 'normal' plyometric programme. As older athletes do not possess the same physiological capabilities as their younger counterparts, at least three to five days of rest should be planned between explosive training sessions. Of course, every athlete has his or her own story, so treat each case individually.

COMMON MISTAKES TO AVOID WITH PLYOMETRICS

Unfortunately many coaches, personal trainers and athletes misunderstand what plyometrics are and how to train correctly. This is normally due to them failing to understand the physiology and training parameters needed to prescribe a progressive plyometric programme correctly. The current trend of performing programmes that are said to be of high intensity and require a person to perform 100 reps in as quick a time as is physically possible is not plyometric and will not make you faster or more explosive. This type of training is both overload and non-explosive with an increased propensity for injury – not something any person wanting to become faster or more explosive should ever consider.

This lack of understanding of the scientific principles of plyometrics can lead to the prescription of incorrect exercises that do not truly take advantage of the stretch-shortening cycle. As mentioned, this current trend of intensity focused workouts often leads to incorrect box jumps heights, especially depth jumps. In this case more, or should we say higher, is not always better. As a result of incorrectly prescribed box heights, athletes end up performing longer contact phases due to the forces absorbed being too great for the athlete to cope with. This longer floor contact time does not elicit a powerful, explosive movement and essentially nullifies the plyometric objective of the training programme. In addition to this, many programmes thought to be plyometric end up becoming conditioning workouts. As mentioned, this new fitness phenomenon of how many reps can you do in a set amount of time or how long does it take you to perform fifty, 100, or many more reps is not plyometric training. Often the mistake of an ill-informed coach or athlete, these types of programmes will never increase an athlete's power and will only put them at risk of potential injury. Volume is normally the first port of call for most coaches when it comes to progressive overload but with plyometrics maintaining quality of movement, intensity and speed of movement should always be on their minds. Athletes should be able to jump on to and off of boxes, which can sometimes be overlooked. Jumping on to boxes with the use of concentric muscle actions through force exertion is easy to prescribe and an athlete gets instant feedback of 'yes I made it' or 'no I didn't'. Coaches should, however, always look to balance out movement patterns when the athlete is physically ready. As well as being able to exert force, an expert well-rounded athlete should be able to absorb it. This is trained through the use of exercises such as depth jumps but only when the athlete is ready.

ARE YOU STRONG ENOUGH FOR PLYOMETRICS?

Through my own research and refinement of training programmes I would suggest that being able to perform twenty reps of body weight exercises such as press-ups, inverted rows, squats, lunges, step-ups, pull-ups, sit-ups and dorsal raises with perfect technique is a good foundation for athletic strength development. It is also a simple precursor to training more explosive movements such as plyometric jumps in place and standing jumps, which place high demand on controlling the body's movements.

There are numerous fundamental movement progression plans that have been developed of late and the following exercises are what we have developed at the Training Shed with coaches Alexa Passingham and Roy Barber. Both these coaches work with developing young athletes in schools between the ages of eleven and fifteen. We have found strong correlations between the ability to complete the following movement progressions for brace, hinge, squat, lunge, push and pull exercises and overall athletic ability in children. I would, however, advise that any athlete undertaking a plyometric programme should be able to complete all the following exercises throughout the

continuum at a 20RM rep range. Developing a good foundation of strength and across multiple planes of motion and different movement patterns will not only develop a functional athlete but one less prone to injury. In turn, this will result in an athlete with more confidence in his or her abilities.

While writing this book, I have had the privilege of conversing with Dr Michael Yessis on multiple occasions. He too has developed a positive training programme based on the principle of 1 × 20RM strength training, which he states has even surprised him as to the effect it is having on athletes. Although this was initially conceived and written for the beginner and high school athlete, Dr Yessis mentioned many of the college coaches using this method are experiencing great gains, more than on a typical high intensity programme. For me, this proves the efficacy of developing solid foundations for any athlete through the development of strength and strength endurance. Obviously the earlier we do this, the more potential that athlete will realize.

Although not essential, being able to complete a 1RM equal to an athlete's bodyweight in push, pull, lunge and squat exercises such as bench press, bench pull, back squat and overhead lunge variations will also greatly enhance any plyometric programme when undertaking higher intensity plyometric drills such as multiple hops and jumps, bounding, box drills and depth jumps. In addition to this, the introduction of Olympic lifting techniques such as the snatch, clean and clean and jerk will enable an athlete to develop sound athletic movements safely with regards to triple extension of the ankles, knees and hips, which are effective during all lower body plyometric drills. This again should be taught by experienced trainers who understand the fundamentals of Olympic lifting techniques, enabling the athlete to progress safely and appropriately.

BRACE EXERCISE PROGRESSIONS

These exercises address greater control of the lower and mid to upper back and shoulders during movement. They are crucial in developing good core control and posture.

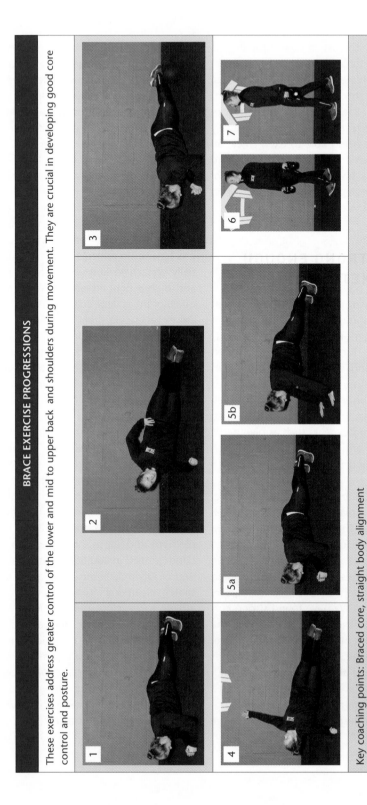

Key coaching points: Braced core, straight body alignment

Table 7 Brace exercises. 1. Front plank; 2. Side plank; 3. Medicine ball front plank; 4. Rotational side plank; 5a and b. Plank builders; 6. Two arm carry; 7. One arm carry.

HINGE EXERCISE PROGRESSIONS

Hip hinge exercises are essential to developing greater athletic strength and athletic. They develop superb flexion and extension strength through the hip joint while ensuring greater spinal control and strength.

Key coaching points: Hinge at the hips, maintain a flat back, weight through the whole foot

Table 8 Hinge exercises. 1. Two leg supine hip bridge; 2. One leg supine hip thrust; 3. Two leg supine hip thrust with BOSU ball; 4. Two leg supine hip thrust with BOSU ball; 5. Kettlebell deadlift; 6. One leg kettlebell deadlift.

SQUAT EXERCISE PROGRESSIONS

An everyday movement pattern that is considered to primarily train the muscles of the legs, hips and back. It also involves the core muscles and upper body.

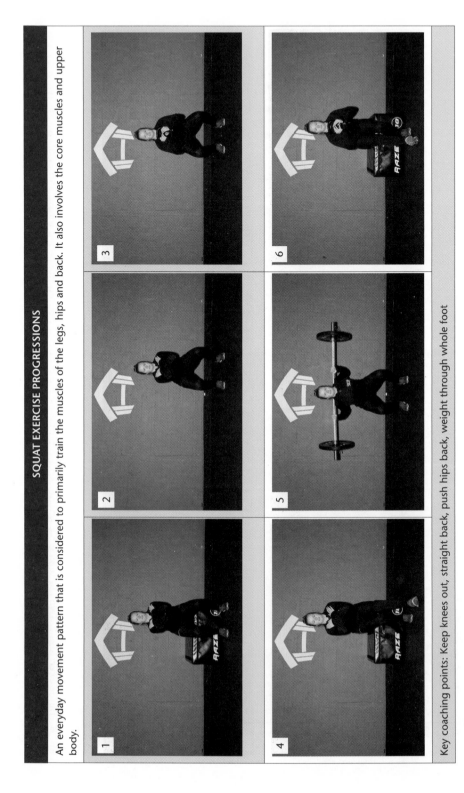

Key coaching points: Keep knees out, straight back, push hips back, weight through whole foot

Table 9   Squat exercises. 1. Bodyweight box squats; 2. Bodyweight air squats; 3. Goblet kettlebell squat; 4. One leg box squat; 5. Loaded barbell back squat; 6. Loaded one leg squat.

LUNGE EXERCISE PROGRESSIONS

Another great lower body exercise that improves the muscles of the lower limbs. Also considered a total body exercise developing core muscles, coordination and proprioception.

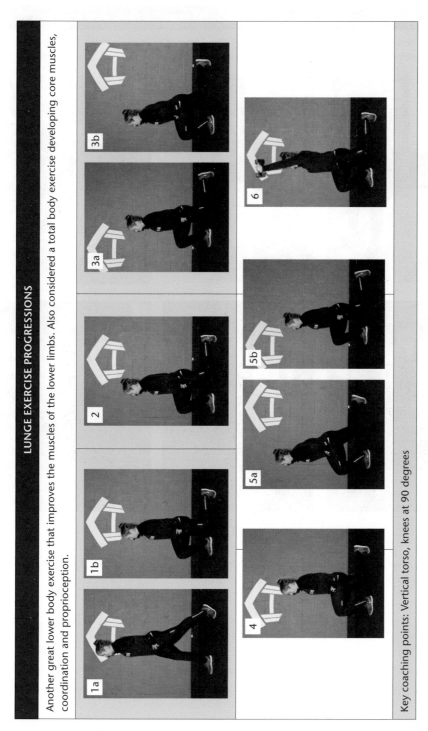

Key coaching points: Vertical torso, knees at 90 degrees

Table 10 Lunge exercises. 1a and b. Split lunge; 2. Forward alternating lunges; 3a and 3b. Forward walking lunges; 4. Reverse alternating lunges; 5a and b. Backward walking lunges; 6. Weighted walking lunges.

PULL EXERCISE PROGRESSIONS

Pull exercises help to develop the muscles of the back, shoulders, biceps and core and are another key movement pattern for developing greater athletic control and posture.

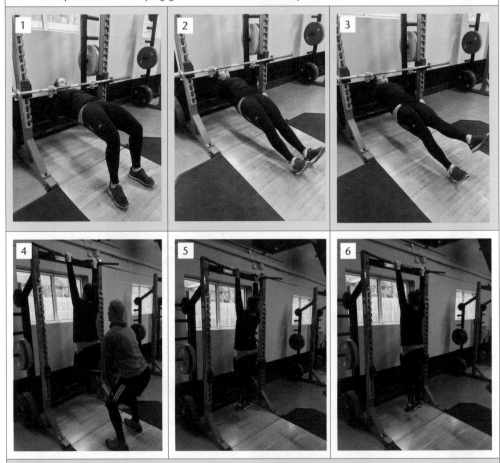

Key coaching points: Pull from elbows, chin over the bar, full extension, braced core.

Table 11 Pull exercises. 1. Bent knee inverted; 2. Straight leg inverted row; 3. One leg inverted row; 4. Assisted pull up; 5. Chin up; 6. Pull up.

PUSH EXERCISE PROGRESSIONS

Push exercises develop muscles of the chest and arms while also developing stability in the shoulders and greater scapular control.

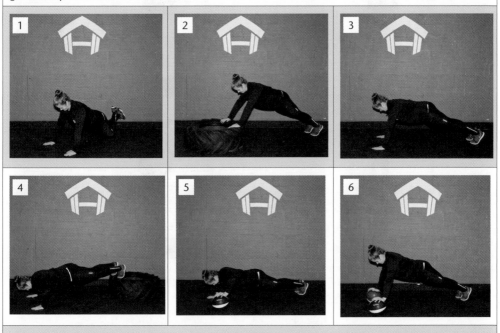

Key coaching points: Straight body alignment, arms tight to torso, controlled movement two up two down

Table 12   Push exercises. 1. Press up on knees; 2. Incline press ups; 3. Press up; 4. Decline press up; 5. One hand med ball press up; 6. Two hand med ball press up.

ASSESSING JUMPING TECHNIQUE

It is always good to analyze technique and with today's technology it is simple to record a video of the following test using your phone or tablet to give you some essential feedback on technique performance. There are some great coaching apps (I use *Coach's Eye* from the App Store) too that will allow you to slow down the video and carry out some in-depth analysis. One tool for assessing and identifying incorrect lower body mechanics in plyometrics is the tuck jump, which interestingly is also seen as a measured way of reducing knee ligament

damage. This repetitive exercise test is usually assessed over a ten-second testing period and will highlight any insufficiencies in technique. The principles of this test should be applied to every plyometric jump when coaching, ensuring correct starting position, peak height and landing mechanics are achieved.

Use the tuck jump athlete checklist to assess your athletes on the tuck jump techniques. Their scores will enable you to programme additional strength work, technique sessions or ensure they are performing the correct level of plyometrics in the simple to complex continuum.

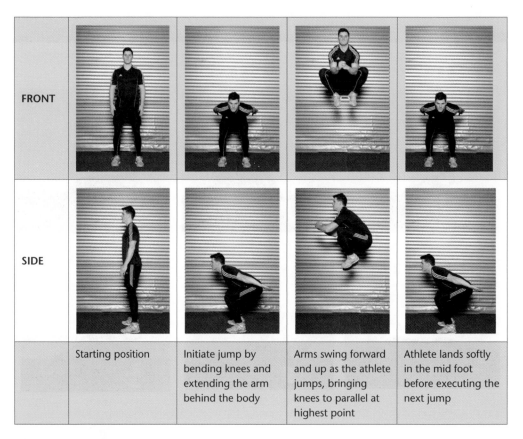

FRONT				
SIDE				
	Starting position	Initiate jump by bending knees and extending the arm behind the body	Arms swing forward and up as the athlete jumps, bringing knees to parallel at highest point	Athlete lands softly in the mid foot before executing the next jump

Table 13   The tuck jump technique.

Athlete		Date	
Sport		D.O.B.	

Starting Jump		Comments
Athlete starts in the athletic position	☐	
Jump is initiated by the legs	☐	
Jump is vertical	☐	
High Point of Tuck Jump		
Thighs reach parallel at peak height of jump	☐	
Thighs reach the same height at peak height of jump	☐	
Athlete retains a straight back with correct head position	☐	
Landing mechanics		
Feet land shoulder width apart – athletic position	☐	
Feet are parallel upon landing	☐	
Feet land at the same time together	☐	
Landing is not heavy	☐	
Multiple Jumps		
Athlete pauses between jumps	☐	
Technique declines over the 10 sec	☐	
Athlete lands inside the test area.	☐	

Table 14   The tuck jump athlete checklist.

WHAT TO LOOK OUT FOR IN THE TUCK JUMP TEST

Starting Jump – To initiate a tuck jump correctly the athlete must first start in the correct athletic position – feet shoulder width apart, pointing forwards with knees slight bent and an upright upper body. The jump must be vertical and initiated by the legs with no excessive arm movement.

High Point of Tuck Jump – Poor core and pelvis control, weak hip flexors and quadriceps muscles can reduce the hip's range of motion and can lead to the athlete's legs not reaching parallel during the high point of the jump. Often imbalanced hip flexors and quadriceps muscles cause one leg to rise higher than the other, which then causes mistimed landing mechanics. Upper body posture can also decline with the athlete flexing forward at the high point to bring the trunk towards the knees. This causes forward movement in the air and reduced high point, which can also lead to wayward landing.

Landing Mechanics – The athlete must land in the same position in which he or she started. Weak gluteal muscles and incorrect landing mechanics can cause the knee to collapse inwards upon landing, which has huge potential for knee ligament damage. Feet can often land too close together reducing the efficiency of the next jump as no power can be transferred through the kinetic chain. Muscle and technique imbalances can cause mistimed landing, which leads to a skipping motion upon the next jump – like a horse doing dressage. One of the most easily recognizable technique flaws is the heavy landing, which causes a loud audible thud. This is normally caused by the athlete landing with straight legs or non-absorbing plyometric landing mechanics causing a forceful 'shock' landing that resonates as increased sound.

Multiple Jumps – Non-plyometric, insufficient rebound mechanics can cause the athlete to pause between jumps, absorbing the plyometric effect. Insufficient muscular endurance and/or jumping technique can cause a decline in quality and thus negate the purpose of jump training. If the athlete is not consistent on landing it can be due to non-vertical take-offs with unwanted forward, backward or sideways movement upon jumping.

5 PLYOMETRIC EQUIPMENT

Plyometrics can be performed anywhere – indoors and outdoors. One important factor is the landing surface used, with grass being one of the best. However, performing plyometrics on rock hard grassy surfaces is not ideal for joints and at the other end of the scale a wet, soggy field can also cause unnecessary injury. Athletics track surfaces are ideally designed for plyometrics but you can also use old school gyms with sprung floors, gymnastic surfaces and matted areas. Using surfaces or mats with too much give can counteract the effects of the plyometric sequence as it prolongs the coupling part, reducing the unloading forces, so ensure your surfaces do not have too great absorbing properties. As a rule of thumb, concrete or asphalt surfaces should be avoided if possible for long periods of training, especially with multiple jump reps and sets. A lot of professional sports clubs are now using a new type of portable surface called the Aerofloor, which enables the safe training of plyometric and rehabilitation exercises.

TRACK SURFACES

Duraflex

Duraflex is not just rubber flooring, it is a 32mm thick premium training flooring system engineered to maximize comfort, durability and functionality. Duraflex's particular construction provides enhanced shock insulation, making it a perfect plyometric surface.

Aerofloor

The Aerofloor is an athletic training platform that uses high specification fabrics and controlled energy return technology. It gives you an efficient energy giving surface through the elastic recoil properties of the fabric. It also has great energy absorbing properties that help reduce the impact on the joints. It can be used for both lower and upper body plyometrics as well as in rehabilitation programmes. Aerofloor provides a ground-breaking surface for the development of plyometric ability and offers a safe and versatile environment to allow more practice with less joint impact.

There are a lot of plyometric drills that do not require any equipment at all. However, the following is a list of equipment that is essential

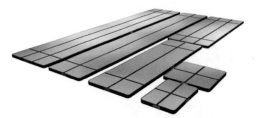

Fig 5.1 The Aerofloor comes in many sizes and can include customized markings.

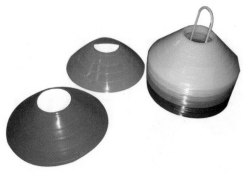

Fig 5.4

if you wish to develop your speed and power to their maximum.

FLOOR MARKING, CONES, LADDERS AND HURDLES

Although you could just jump in the air, having a physical barrier or guide is a great way to focus the mind and ensure you are jumping the correct heights and distances. Floor markings, whether in the shape of grids, hexagons or ladders are great for plyometric assessments drills and ensuring correct landing positions. You could use the lane lines of an athletics track if you don't have the luxury of fancy floor

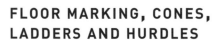

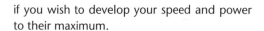

Fig 5.2

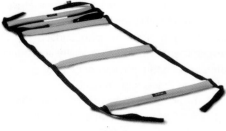

Fig 5.3

markings or even masking tape. Cones should be 8–24in in height. The less experienced plyometric athlete should stick to foam barriers for obvious reasons. Be creative and place wooden dowels on cones or stack up some Airex balance pads.

PLYOMETRIC BOXES AND PLATFORMS

There are many different types of plyometric boxes available but a strong platform box or plywood box is usually great for vertical, horizontal and depth jumping, The RAZE wooden three-in-one plyo box used in this book has three heights in one box – 20in, 24in and 30in. Boxes need to range in height from 6–48in depending on the athlete's ability, and non-slip surfaces are essential for safety. Stackable boxes allow for varying heights and can be stored easily. Soft plyometric boxes are great for beginners and having the advantage of being able to stack them gives you a great progression option as the athlete develops his or her jumping power. The fantastic and incredibly versatile soft plyo boxes used in this book are foam-covered with a hard-wearing, wipe clean vinyl. They offer a soft but stable landing surface that reduces stress on joints, with no danger of shin damage if you miss a jump. Boxes can be used individually or attached securely together to allow many variations in

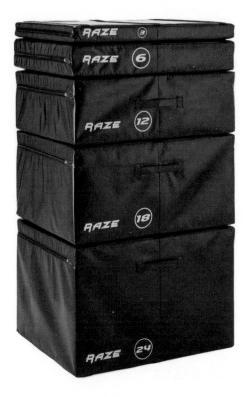

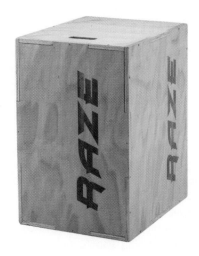

Fig 5.7

Fig 5.5 Soft Plyo Boxes available in: 3in (7.5cm), 6in (15cm), 12in (30cm), 18in (45cm), 24in (60cm) heights – Large landing area of 90cm × 75cm, Covered in wipe clean vinyl. Velcro the boxes together for extra height.

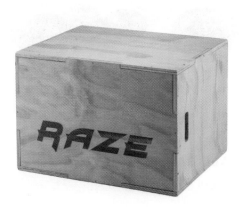

Fig 5.8

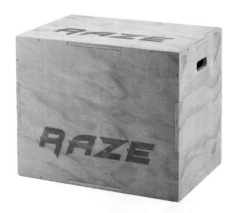

Fig 5.6

height up to a maximum of 160cm (5ft 3in), which should keep you going for a while! They are also light enough to move around your training space easily, making them a great piece of kit for any athlete.

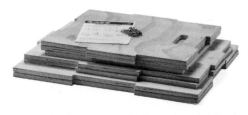

Fig 5.9 The three-in-one plyo box – three heights in one box: 20in, 24in and 30in.

MED BALLS

Used in both upper and lower body plyometric exercises, medicine balls are the perfect tool for developing speed and power. Make sure you get a ball that can handle being thrown around, like the med ball pictured. Medicine balls with grip handles are great for jumping and throwing drills. They are available in 4kg to 10kg weights (see red below). The Raze medicine ball used in this book has a unique construction and high-grip, textured finish, making it perfect for throws and catches. The RAZE dual grip medicine ball features two moulded handles, allowing you to hold it in different ways and so add more specificity to your plyometric drills and diversity to your workouts.

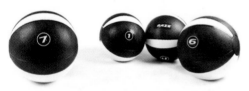

Fig. 5.10 Med balls are available from 4kg to 10kg in 1kg increments.

WALL BALLS

The wall ball is a great sport-specific training tool. It is made from high quality textiles with double-stitched seams throughout. This highly durable yet soft construction makes it suitable for all user abilities and fitness levels by reducing the chances of impact injuries when thrown forcefully and then caught. Lighter wall balls can be used for traditional core strengthening exercises such as weighted sit-ups and throws and Russian twists, but also in the early stages of rehabilitation and with smaller athletes. The heavier wall balls are to be used for carries, loading drills, explosive throws during power development sessions and in conditioning workouts, making them a must for any serious training facility where steady progres-

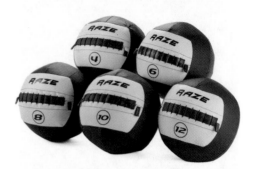

Fig. 5.11 Wall balls are available from 4kg to 12kg in 2kg increments.

sion is required. The great thing about the wall ball is that it has the same 36cm (14in) diameter whatever the weight, so you can progress up and down the weights without having to worry about altering your technique.

SLAM BALLS

It's not a good idea to slam a med ball, well unless you've got deep pockets! Being slammed with power will have a detrimental effect and nine times out of ten they will split. I would recommend a slam ball because, as the name suggests, you can pretty much do what you want with it. This training tool is the ideal companion to traditional medicine balls and wall balls as it is designed to be slammed – against walls, into floors… pretty much anywhere. We tested slam balls in the Training Shed for Indigo Fitness because we split all our med balls doing plyometric drills and we can honestly say that, so far, we have not broken any slam balls.

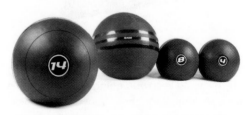

Fig. 5.12 Slam balls are available in 4kg, 6kg, 8kg, 10kg, 12kg and 14kg.

WEIGHTED WEARABLES

You should never wear extra weight for prolonged periods of time when performing plyometric training. However, training research has shown that adding additional kilograms through a weighted vest such as the raptor vest can enhance your plyometric training. A vest that allows you to add progressive and changeable loads that fits snug to the body is recommended in order to keep the exercise truly plyometric. You can also use ankle weights and belts to the same effect but always ensure you do not overload and alter your technique.

STEPS, STAIRS AND PARK BENCHES

All of these are accessible to everyone and, of course, are free. However, make sure they are safe and sufficiently engineered to take your body weight and more. They weren't designed to be jumped on and off so do not use them without checking their viability properly.

THINGS TO REMEMBER

- Avoid concrete or asphalt surfaces, especially for long periods of plyometric training.
- Ensure your landing surface has some give in it to protect your joints.
- Soft barriers and plyometric boxes should be used by beginner athletes.
- Always check the structure of steps and benches as they were not designed for jumping.

6 | PLYOMETRIC TRAINING – THE WARM-UP

Plyometrics are very demanding on the body and as such should never be performed 'cold'. A thorough warm-up is needed to ensure the stretch-shortening cycle is fully engaged to give maximal power output. A tight or cold muscle is more susceptible to injury in any activity but due to the rapid movement of plyometric exercises this potential is greatly increased. A warm-up's primary purpose is to ready the athlete for the workload they are to perform in the main part of their planned session. Therefore, a warm-up should start slowly and build in intensity over a period of time. It is generally considered that fifteen to twenty minutes is a good length of time for a warm-up. However, you could say it is down to the athlete to know when they are truly ready.

The purpose of a warm-up is to:

• Increase body temperature
• Increase heart rate and blood flow
• Increase breathing rate
• Increase elasticity of muscular system
• Activate the neuromuscular system
• Increase mental alertness.

A properly designed warm-up should start with some light mobility work and/or foam rolling. Foam rolling, or to give its proper name self-myofascial release, is a relatively cheap and easy way to help maintain healthy muscle function. Its primary purpose is to release any muscular tight spots or trigger points that might impinge on the muscle's ability to contract efficiently. It is known as foam rolling simply due to the piece of equipment used but, depending on your pain threshold, you can use pretty much anything including a tennis ball, golf ball, lacrosse ball or even a piece of drain-pipe. The process will help to stimulate blood flow while increasing muscle elasticity. When used for between five to ten minutes prior to beginning your active warm-up, self-myofascial release will help ensure your muscles are free from knots and improve their ability to establish proper movement patterns and maintain good blood flow. Performing foam rolling after activity has also been scientifically proven to reduce post-exercise muscle fatigue, helping to maintain healthy functional muscles and improve performance.

SELF-MYOFASCIAL RELEASE (AKA FOAM ROLLING)

Table 15 shows you ten simple self-myofascial release exercises that will help to maintain

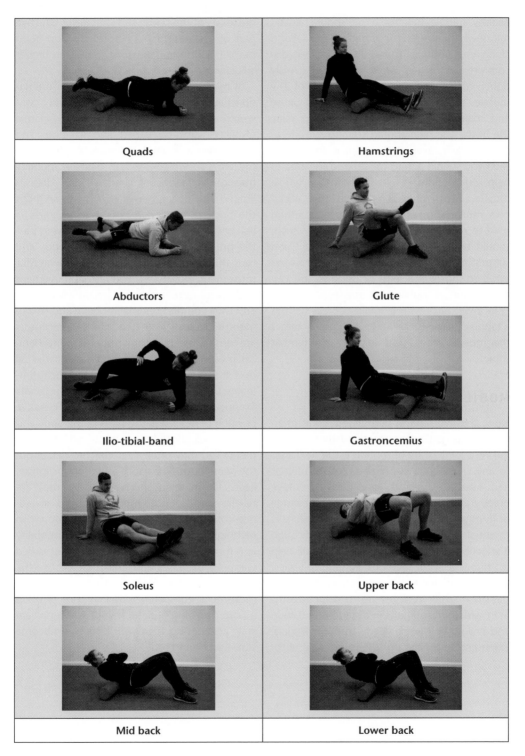

Table 15 Self-myofascial release exercises.

healthy muscle function. You should always roll slowly, aiming to for about 1in per second along your muscle. You will feel a slight discomfort (or maybe more if you are really tight) when rolling over tight areas of the muscle. When this occurs, you should pause and maintain deep breathing to help relax the body. The pain should start to subside as the muscle relaxes. If the pain is too much, then you should aim to roll around the area to help reduce tightness throughout the whole muscle. Self-myofascial release is not about how much pain you can take, it is a method used to reduce muscle tightness and, as such, should be used sensibly to alleviate pain and stiffness rather than cause it. You should always avoid rolling over a joint or bone as this can cause injury. I would also advise not rolling your lower back with a smaller object such as a tennis or lacrosse ball in order to really target the muscles and avoid injuring the lumbar spine.

MOBILITY WARM-UP

Now that you have completed your foam rolling it is generally considered that increasing your joint range of motion is the next step to any warm-up. With regards to plyometrics you need to prepare your body to move quickly and with force, so having great range of motion across the main joint movers is essential. Mobility can be increased through a selection of exercises and drills that will help to stimulate your nervous system, muscles, tendons and joints to ensure you make the transition safely from resting to session-ready. Start with joint rotations in a standing position and ensure you work slowly through flexing, extending and rotating where possible all of the joints of the body. This simple yet effective part of a warm-up will help to develop good mobility and prepare your joints for higher velocity movements.

It might surprise you to learn but coordination happens in the brain, not the body. So I would always suggest you keep your dynamic mobility warm-up varied and exciting. You only have a limited number of joints but the ways in which you can develop mobility through variations of exercises and drills is limited only by your creativity. The brain maps the body through networks that organize its ability to move, so the bigger the moving part the greater the sensory motor demands and thus the need for more efficient pathways for movement. However, if you restrict movement in these joints the pathways become less active and thus you find optimal mobility and movement difficult or restricted. Mechanoreceptors are sensory receptors that respond to mechanical pressure or distortion and are located all over the body. When movement or touch stimulates these receptors, proprioception occurs. Proprioception is the sense of the relative position of neighbouring parts of the body and strength of effort being employed in movement. You may often hear coaches talk about the need for good balance and proprioception, especially in team sports. Basically, they are talking about good movement and awareness of movement, which is also known as technique. So, to truly develop good mobility and movement it is recommended that varied warm-up exercises and drills that expose the body to greater degrees of movement and movement competency will in turn develop a better moving athlete. If your warm-ups are stale and boring then your body will become stale and boring too!

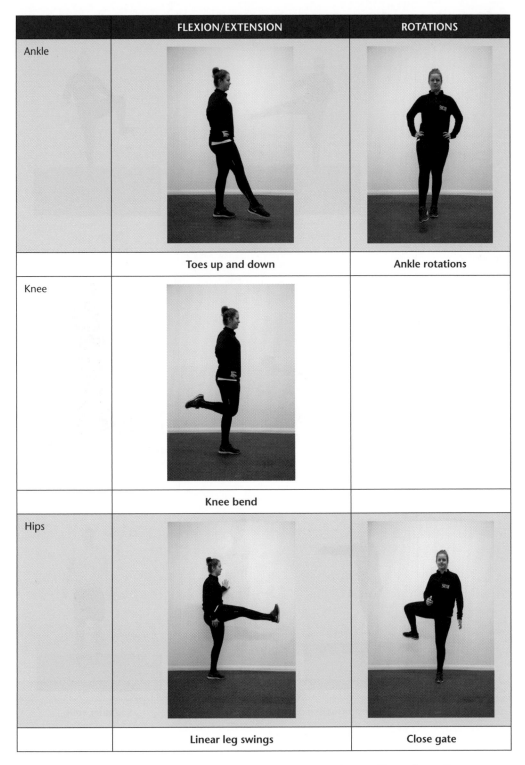

	FLEXION/EXTENSION	ROTATIONS
Ankle	Toes up and down	Ankle rotations
Knee	Knee bend	
Hips	Linear leg swings	Close gate

Table 16   Joint and body mobility exercises. Start from the ground up (ankles to fingers!) × ten reps each movement (no more than four to five minutes in total time).

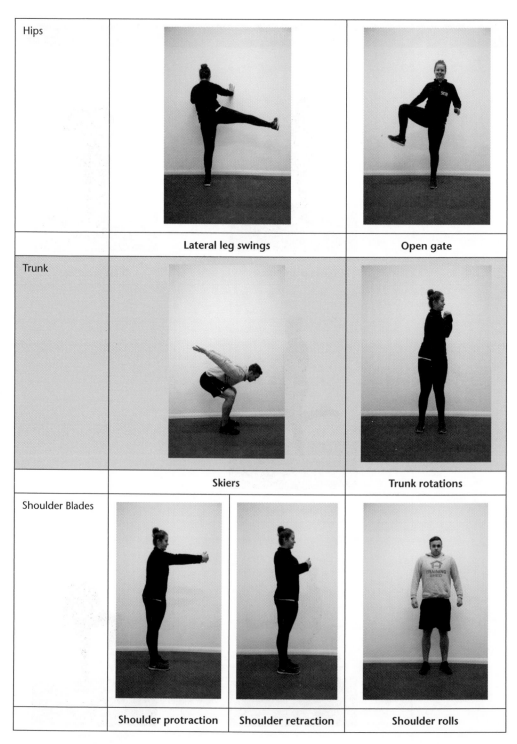

Hips	Lateral leg swings	Open gate
Trunk	Skiers	Trunk rotations
Shoulder Blades	Shoulder protraction / Shoulder retraction	Shoulder rolls

Table 16 *Continued.*

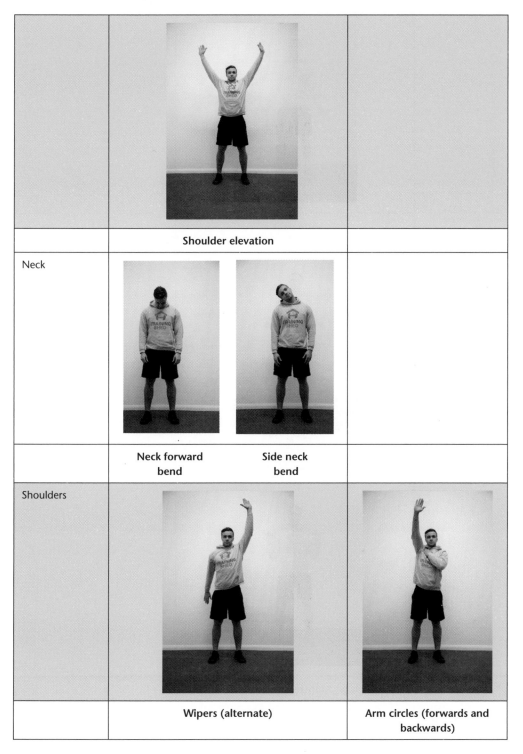

	Shoulder elevation	
Neck	**Neck forward bend** **Side neck bend**	
Shoulders	**Wipers (alternate)**	**Arm circles (forwards and backwards)**

Table 16 *Continued.*

Elbows	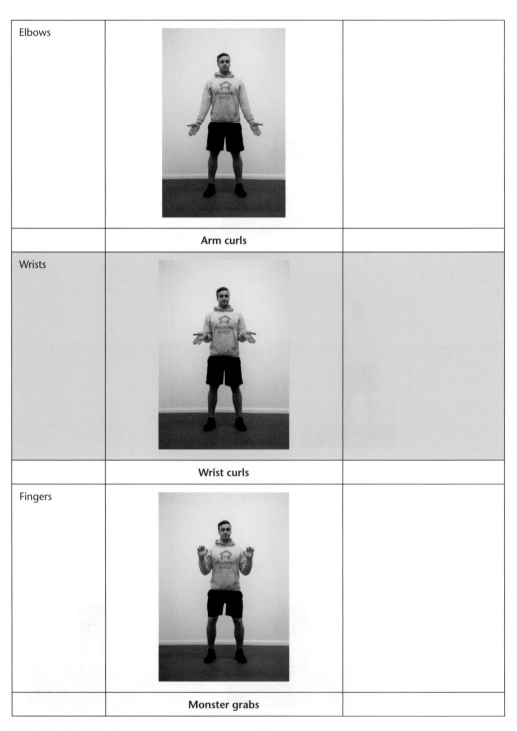	
	Arm curls	
Wrists		
	Wrist curls	
Fingers		
	Monster grabs	

Table 16 *Continued.*

DYNAMIC MOBILITY DRILLS

Following the increase in joint range of motion the next stage would be to use a few drills that help to increase joint mobility and muscle elasticity while increasing heart rate and body temperature. The following drills are all performed over a distance of 5–20m and carried out at a low to medium intensity.

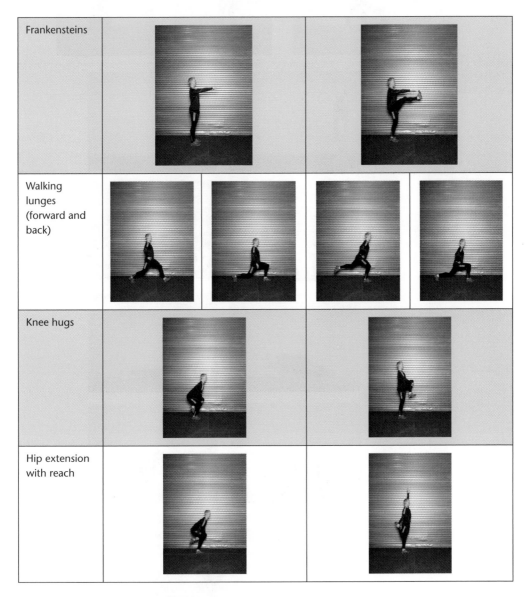

Frankensteins		
Walking lunges (forward and back)		
Knee hugs		
Hip extension with reach		

Table 17   Dynamic mobility drills.

Sumo squats with rotation	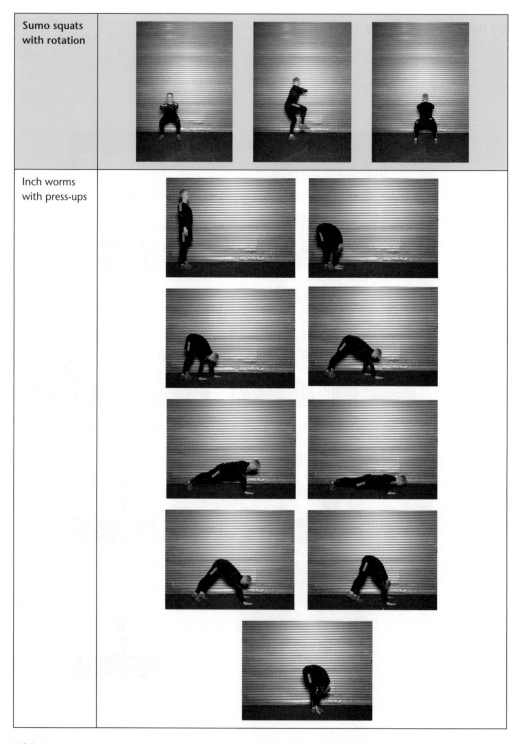
Inch worms with press-ups	

Table 17 *Continued.*

Spiderman

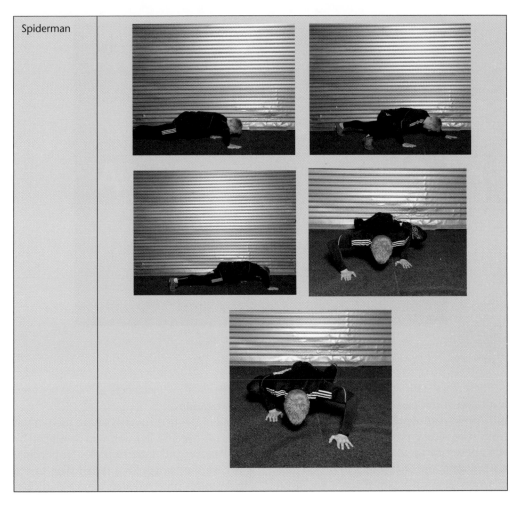

Table 17 *Continued.*

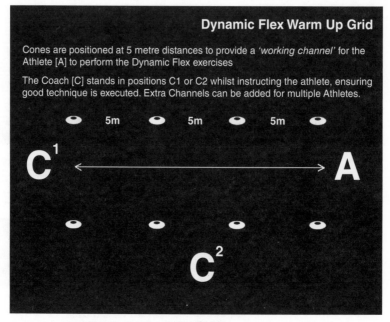

Fig 6.1 Dynamic flex warm-up grid.

These days static stretching for a warm-up is a thing of the past and the new buzz term is dynamic warm-up. Dynamic warm-ups have been scientifically proven to increase an athlete's power by up to 30 per cent over that of a static warm-up. So it stands to reason that a dynamic warm-up is best practice not just for plyometrics but any form of performance exercise or sport where maximal velocity muscle contractions occur. Some advocates of static stretching say it reduces injury, however a study of army recruits by an Australian physiotherapist has proved this not to be the case.

Physiotherapist Pope instructed half his recruits to warm up with static stretching and the other half to warm up with dynamic stretching over the course of a year and found no differences in incidences of injury between the two groups.

One of the best routines I have used in the past is the dynamic flex warm-up developed by Alan Pearson SAQ International. The principle is to take the body from a rested state to the physiological state required for the participation in the main session that follows, through the use of dynamic flex exercises that:

- increase body temperature
- increase heart rate and blood flow
- increase breathing rate
- increase elasticity of the muscular system
- activate the neuromuscular system
- increase mental alertness.

DYNAMIC FLEX WARM-UPS

Traditionally used in team sports such as football, hockey, rugby and netball, this routine uses a 20m × 20m grid and is a great way of warming up any number of athletes. The athletes work forwards for 20m with the coach positioned at the front of the grid so everyone can hear and see the drill cues. Maintaining a forward facing position, he or she then works backwards in the grid. The warm-up starts slowly, building to a session specific intensity. Each dynamic flex warm-up can and should be different and does not have to follow a set drills pattern. However, it generally starts at the foot/ankle and works through the body's joints before engaging in some high explosive all body movements such as short sprinting. The following table shows some examples of exercises and drills used in a dynamic flex warm-up.

WALKING ON THE BALLS OF THE FEET	
To improve ankle mobility, stretch shins and increase balance and coordination	
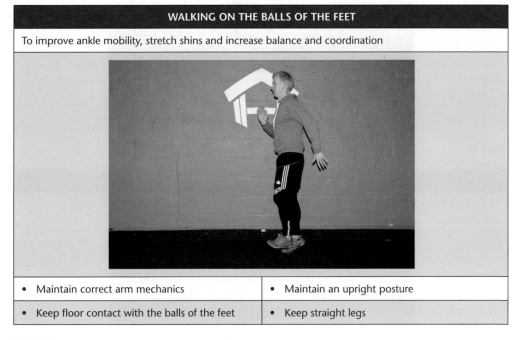	
• Maintain correct arm mechanics	• Maintain an upright posture
• Keep floor contact with the balls of the feet	• Keep straight legs

Table 18

57

ANKLE FLICKS
To stretch calves and improve ankle mobility. To improve balance, coordination and rhythm of movement. To prepare good foot-to-floor contact

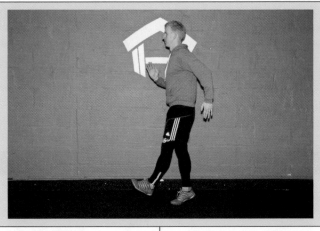

• Practise on the spot before moving forwards	• Maintain an upright posture
• Keep floor contact with the balls of the feet	• Keep straight legs

Table 19

SMALL SKIPS
To improve lower leg dynamic mobility. To develop positive lower leg mechanics, balance and coordination

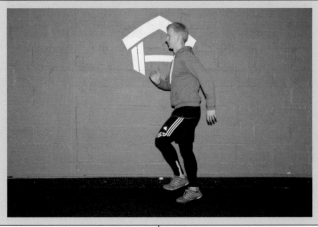

• Knee to be raised to approx 45-55 degrees	• Maintain an upright posture
• Keep floor contact with the balls of the feet	• Work off the balls of the feet.

Table 20

WIDE SKIPS
To increase hip and ankle mobility. To improve balance, coordination and rhythm

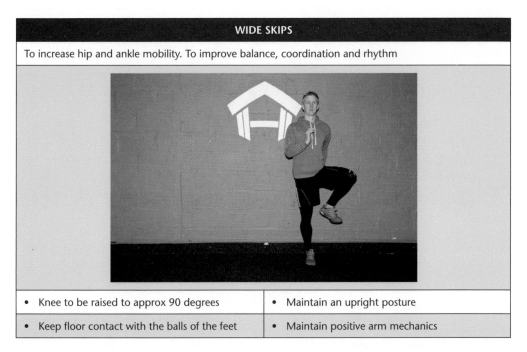

• Knee to be raised to approx 90 degrees	• Maintain an upright posture
• Keep floor contact with the balls of the feet	• Maintain positive arm mechanics

Table 21

SINGLE KNEE, DEAD-LEG LIFT
To improve hip mobility, to promote positive knee lift and running mechanics

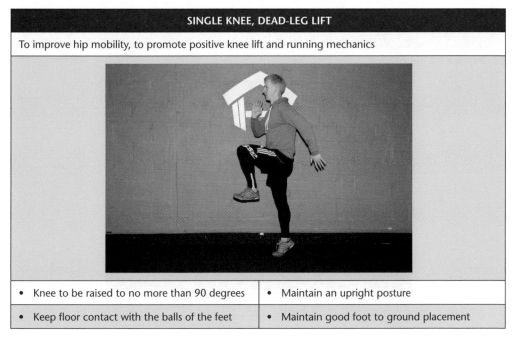

• Knee to be raised to no more than 90 degrees	• Maintain an upright posture
• Keep floor contact with the balls of the feet	• Maintain good foot to ground placement

Table 22

HIGH KNEE-LIFT SKIP
To improve hip mobility and range of motion

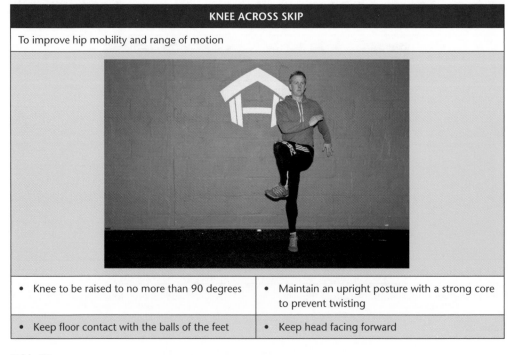

• Knee to be raised to no more than 90 degrees	• Maintain an upright posture with a strong core to prevent twisting
• Keep floor contact with the balls of the feet	• Keep head facing forward

Table 23

KNEE ACROSS SKIP
To improve hip mobility and range of motion

• Knee to be raised to no more than 90 degrees	• Maintain an upright posture with a strong core to prevent twisting
• Keep floor contact with the balls of the feet	• Keep head facing forward

Table 24

LATERAL RUNNING
To improve coordination and balance. Promote positive foot contact timing

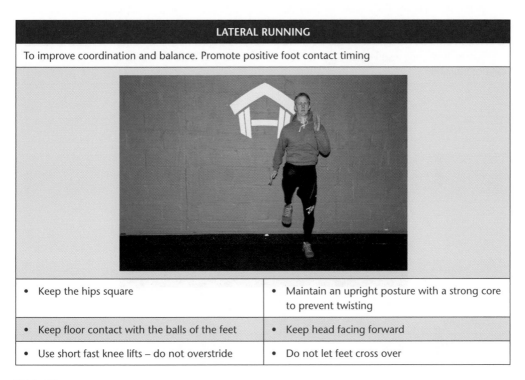

• Keep the hips square	• Maintain an upright posture with a strong core to prevent twisting
• Keep floor contact with the balls of the feet	• Keep head facing forward
• Use short fast knee lifts – do not overstride	• Do not let feet cross over

Table 25

KNEE OUT SKIP
To improve hip mobility and range of motion through abductor/adductors

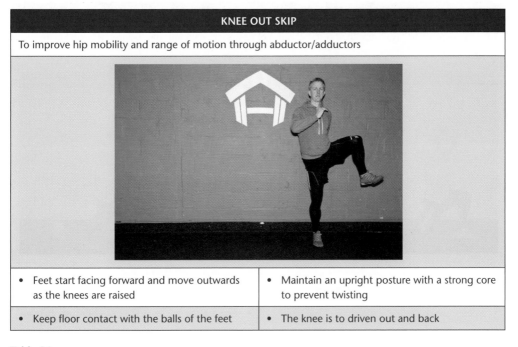

• Feet start facing forward and move outwards as the knees are raised	• Maintain an upright posture with a strong core to prevent twisting
• Keep floor contact with the balls of the feet	• The knee is to driven out and back

Table 26

RUSSIAN WALK
To increase hamstring flexibility and hip mobility. Development of ankle stabilization through balance and coordination

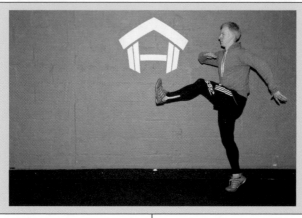

• Lift the knee first, before extending the hamstring	• Maintain an upright posture
• Work off the balls of the feet	• Keep the hips square

Table 27

WALKING LUNGES FORWARD AND BACKWARD
To increase hip mobility, strength and stabilization of posterior chain and hip flexors. Develop balance and coordination

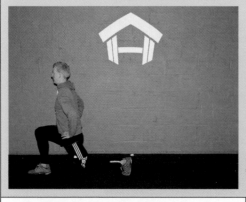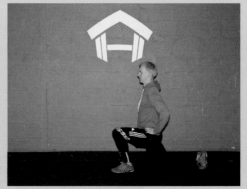

• Try to walk the lunge without standing with feet together to recover as you move forward.	• Maintain an upright posture
• Keep the hips square	• Practise the backwards lunges because they are difficult!

Table 28

SIDE LUNGE
To increase hip mobility, strength and stabilization of posterior chain and hip flexors. Develop balance and coordination

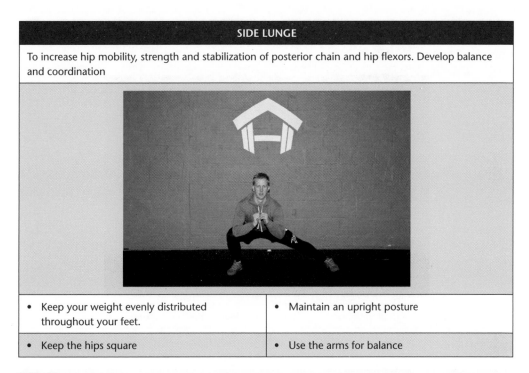

• Keep your weight evenly distributed throughout your feet.	• Maintain an upright posture
• Keep the hips square	• Use the arms for balance

Table 29

HURDLE WALK
To increase hip range of motion. Develop balance and coordination

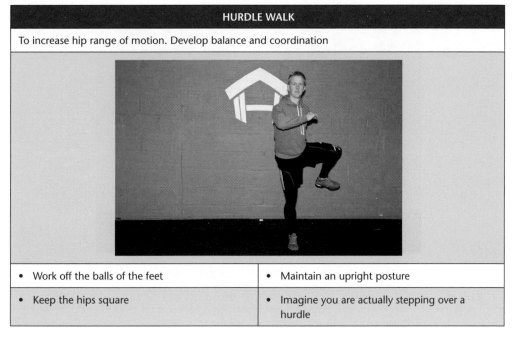

• Work off the balls of the feet	• Maintain an upright posture
• Keep the hips square	• Imagine you are actually stepping over a hurdle

Table 30

WALKING HAMSTRING	
To increase hamstring mobility	
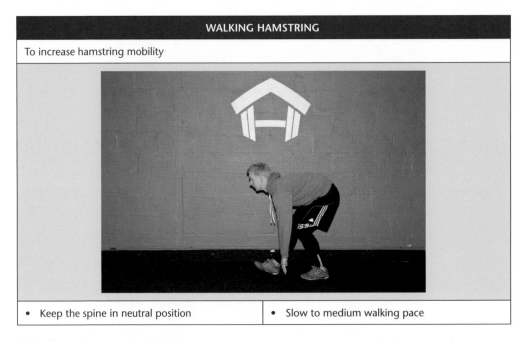	
• Keep the spine in neutral position	• Slow to medium walking pace

Table 31

HAMSTRINGS BUTTOCK KICKS	
To promote good lower leg mechanics	
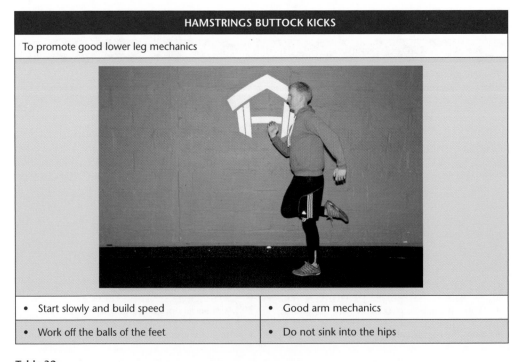	
• Start slowly and build speed	• Good arm mechanics
• Work off the balls of the feet	• Do not sink into the hips

Table 32

CARIOCA
To improve hip/trunk mobility and speed of movement

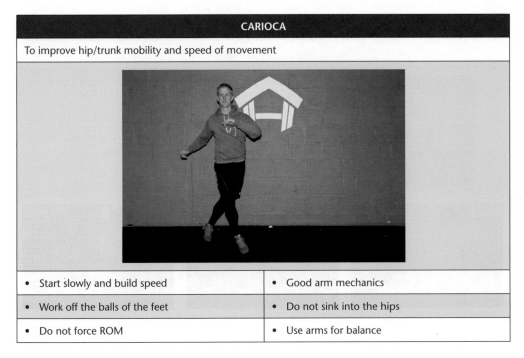

• Start slowly and build speed	• Good arm mechanics
• Work off the balls of the feet	• Do not sink into the hips
• Do not force ROM	• Use arms for balance

Table 33

SPEED AND MOVEMENT DRILLS

As well as being great movement teaching drills in their own right, the following drills can be used in the last minutes of a warm-up to prepare the athlete mentally for the explosive training drills of the main session. The use of drills is not only enjoyable but plays a large part in developing sound movement and speed. The trick here is to be creative and never use the same drill over and over, week in, week out. It is also not advised to use this time as a teaching period for these drills. Only use the drills that the athletes feel comfortable with and show competency otherwise you will find this part of the warm-up decreasing in intensity and turning into a coaching session. The idea is to pick a few drills and do them for three to five minutes to help increase body temperature, heart rate and mental and physical alertness.

Sprints with Varied Starts

This simple sprinting drill can be performed over 5–30m. By varying the starts, you will ensure the athlete is not only warmed up fully but able to react to start commands from obscure positions. This will test the body and reactions of the athlete. Some examples of start positions include standing, kneeling, one-knee kneeling, sitting, lying face down, lying face up and starting with your back to the coach so you can react only on voice command. Have fun with these and be creative.

Hurdle Drills

These drills are great for warming up as they focus on good mechanics and range of motion. Arm and lift (knee) mechanics are important in most sports and ensuring good technique in your warm-up through the use of these drills will reinforce good running mechanics. Only use these drills once they have been perfected.

SINGLE LEG RUN

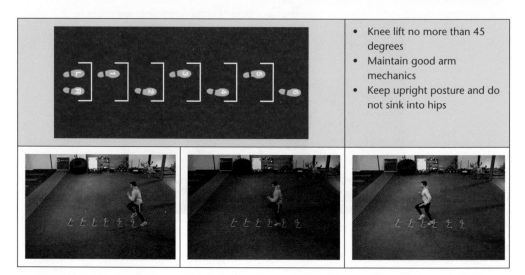

- Knee lift no more than 45 degrees
- Maintain good arm mechanics
- Keep upright posture and do not sink into hips

Table 34

DOUBLE LEG RUN

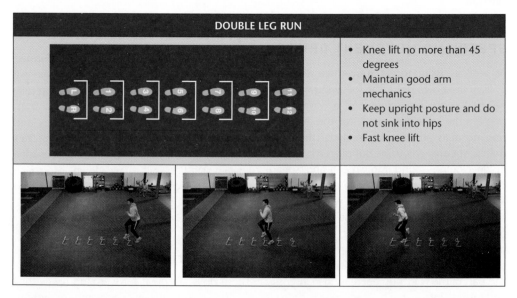

- Knee lift no more than 45 degrees
- Maintain good arm mechanics
- Keep upright posture and do not sink into hips
- Fast knee lift

Table 35

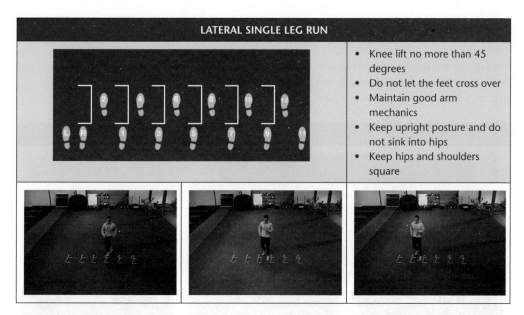

LATERAL SINGLE LEG RUN

- Knee lift no more than 45 degrees
- Do not let the feet cross over
- Maintain good arm mechanics
- Keep upright posture and do not sink into hips
- Keep hips and shoulders square

Table 36

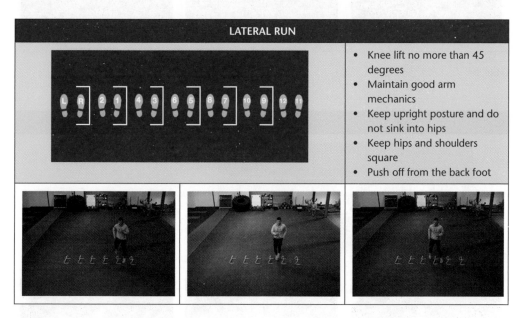

LATERAL RUN

- Knee lift no more than 45 degrees
- Maintain good arm mechanics
- Keep upright posture and do not sink into hips
- Keep hips and shoulders square
- Push off from the back foot

Table 37

Ladder Drills

These drills are to be performed at a higher intensity to the hurdle drills. They will prepare the body for faster more explosive movements, ensuring the neural pathways are awake.

Ladder drills also help to focus the mind. These drills should not be used in a warm-up until they are perfected as they will not get the desired effect if practised at less than 100 per cent intensity.

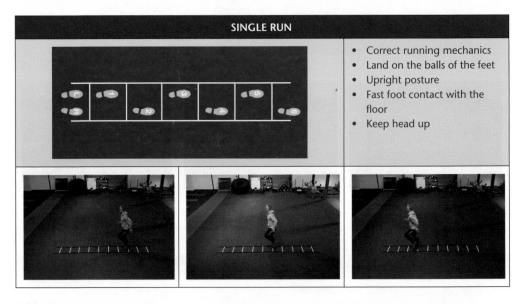

Table 38

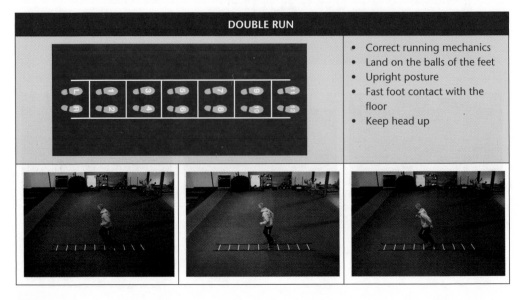

Table 39

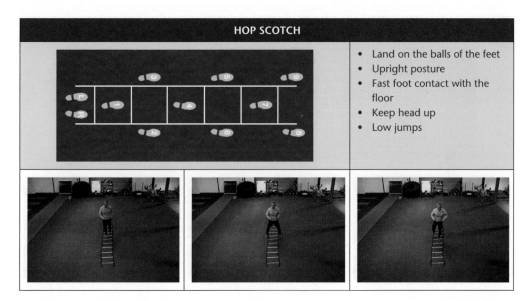

Table 40

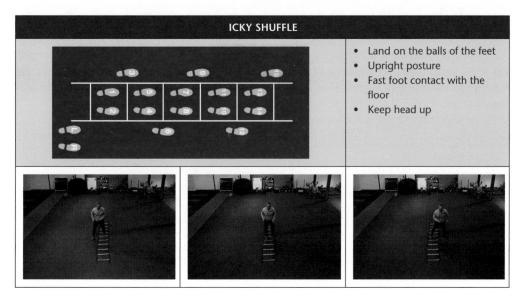

Table 41

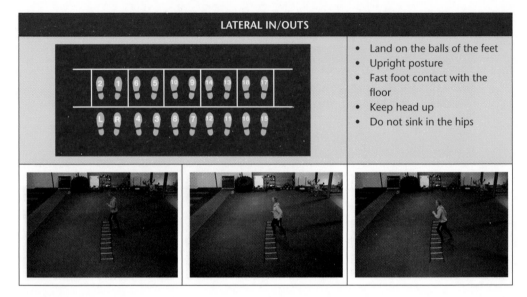

LATERAL IN/OUTS

- Land on the balls of the feet
- Upright posture
- Fast foot contact with the floor
- Keep head up
- Do not sink in the hips

Table 42

Cone Drills

Agility drills such as these are great for improving the speed and power of your player. However, they are also a great way to spice up your warm-ups. The different movement patterns observed in these drills will ensure any athlete is prepared fully for plyometric training. Stay close to the cones and run as fast as you can. I would recommend only performing three to six reps (1min rest) of one or a mixture of the drills below before undertaking your main plyometric work.

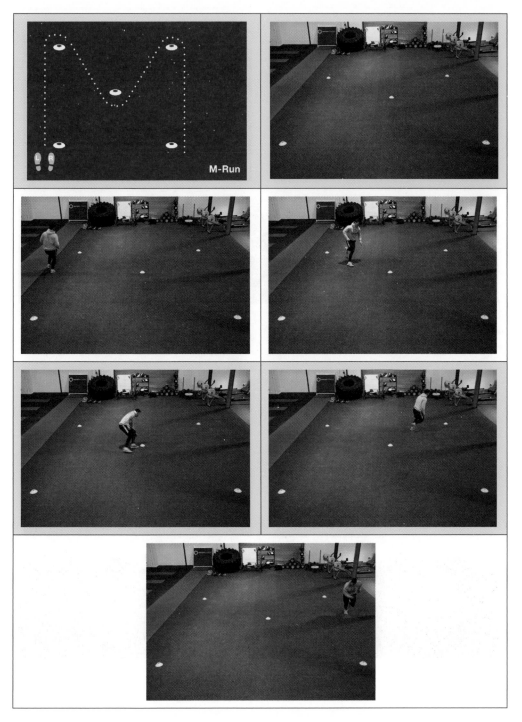

Table 43

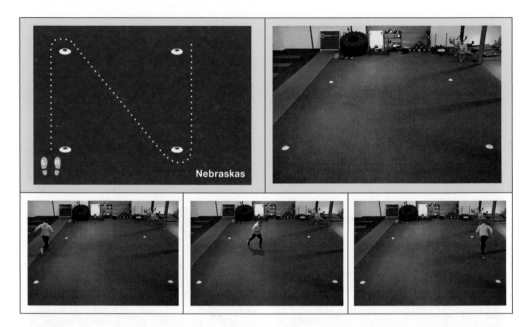

Table 44

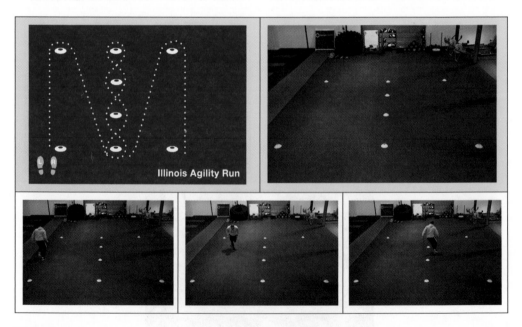

Table 45

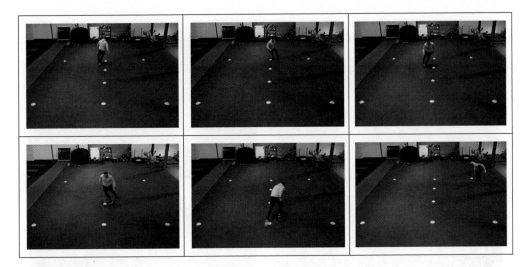

Table 45   *Continued.*

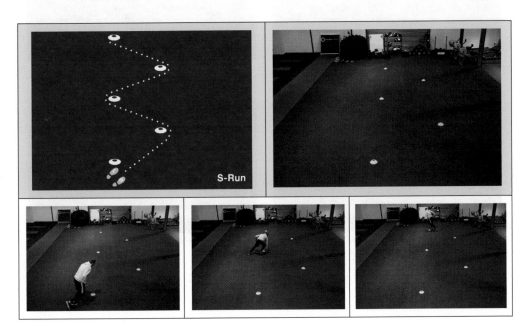

Table 46

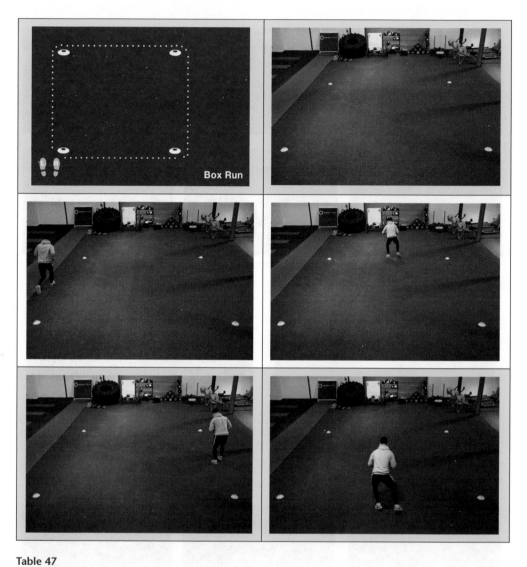

Box Run

Table 47

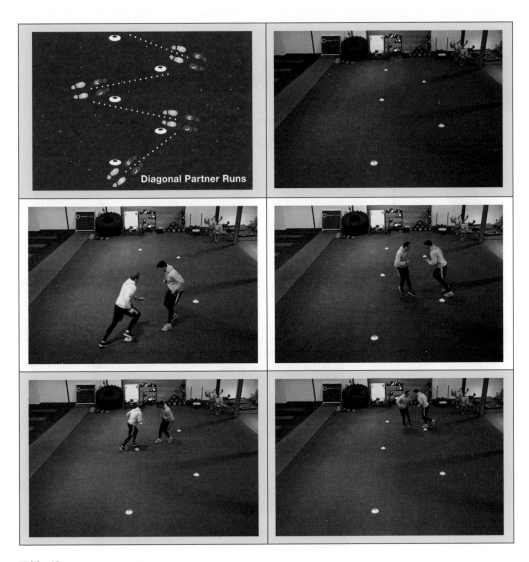

Diagonal Partner Runs

Table 48

THINGS TO REMEMBER

- Self-myofascial release is not about how much pain you can take. It is a method used to reduce muscle tightness and as such should be used sensibly to alleviate pain and stiffness rather than cause it.
- Use speed and movement drills that athletes are competent at in the warm-up. If they are not able to keep the intensity then it will defeat the purpose of this part of the routine. Keep drill teaching to main session content.
- Make sure all your athletes understand the importance of correct mechanics over intensity. The athletic position is vitally important and should be practised.

7 | PLYOMETRIC EXERCISES

JUMPS IN PLACE EXERCISES

Exercise	Two foot ankle hop.
Images	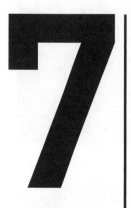
Equipment	None
Start	Start in an upright position with feet together.
Action	From a standing position, and without using your arms, spring upwards using only your ankles. Repeat for the required number of reps.

Table 49

Exercise	Two foot twist hops.
Images	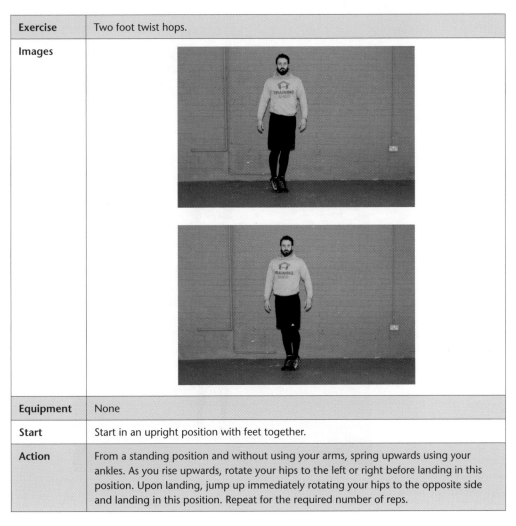
Equipment	None
Start	Start in an upright position with feet together.
Action	From a standing position and without using your arms, spring upwards using your ankles. As you rise upwards, rotate your hips to the left or right before landing in this position. Upon landing, jump up immediately rotating your hips to the opposite side and landing in this position. Repeat for the required number of reps.

Table 50

Exercise	Squat jump.
Images	
Equipment	None
Start	Start in a standing position with your hands behind your head.
Action	Bend your knees into a squat position and explode immediately upwards in a vertical jump, ensuring full triple extension of the hips, knees and ankles. Land in a squat position. This drill can be a single or multiple response drill. Maintain your hands behind your head throughout.

Table 51

Exercise	Rocket jump.
Images	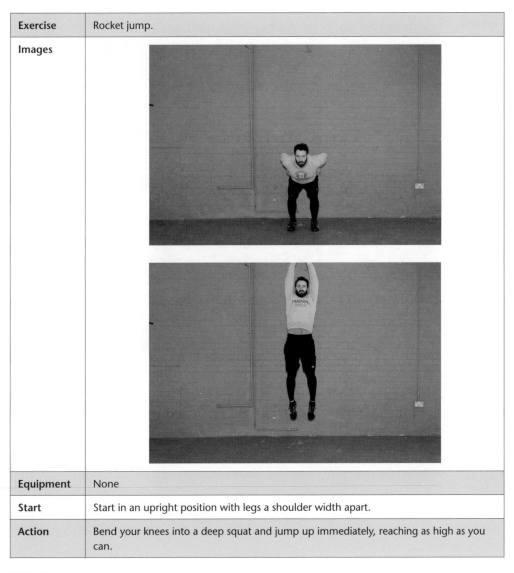
Equipment	None
Start	Start in an upright position with legs a shoulder width apart.
Action	Bend your knees into a deep squat and jump up immediately, reaching as high as you can.

Table 52

Exercise	Star jump.
Images	
Equipment	None
Start	Start in an upright position.
Action	Using your arms and legs, squat down and jump up immediately. As you jump fully, extend your arms and legs out diagonally into a 'star' position.

Table 53

Exercise	Side to side ankle hop.
Images	
Equipment	None.
Start	Start in an upright position on one leg. This leg should be on the opposite side of the body to which you will be hopping laterally.
Action	Bend your knee slightly to allow your ankle to flex. Hop sideways, landing on your other leg. Repeat this, hopping from side to side for the required reps.

Table 54

Exercise	Side to side single leg ankle hop.
Images	
Equipment	None.
Start	Start in an upright position on one leg. This leg should be on the opposite side of the body to which you will be hopping laterally.
Action	Bend your knee slightly to allow your ankle to flex. Hop sideways landing on the same foot. Repeat this, hopping from side to side for the required reps.

Table 55

Exercise	Tuck jump with butt kick.
Images	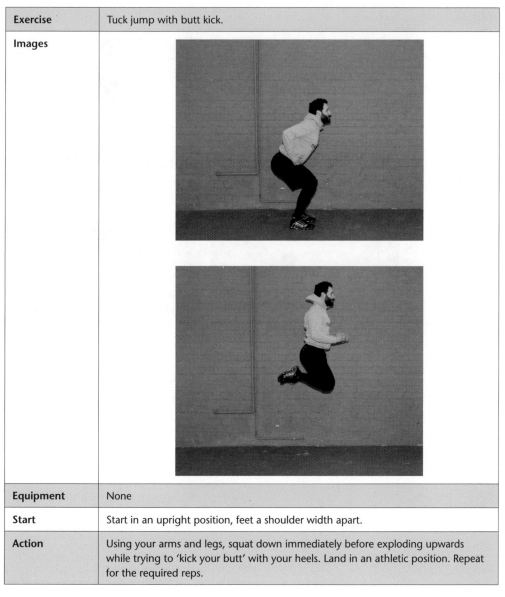
Equipment	None
Start	Start in an upright position, feet a shoulder width apart.
Action	Using your arms and legs, squat down immediately before exploding upwards while trying to 'kick your butt' with your heels. Land in an athletic position. Repeat for the required reps.

Table 56

Exercise	Tuck jump.
Images	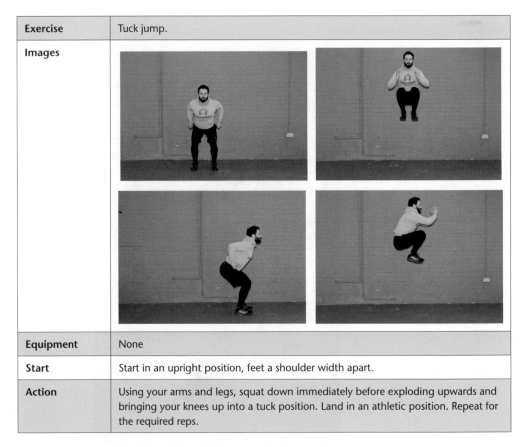
Equipment	None
Start	Start in an upright position, feet a shoulder width apart.
Action	Using your arms and legs, squat down immediately before exploding upwards and bringing your knees up into a tuck position. Land in an athletic position. Repeat for the required reps.

Table 57

Exercise	Split squat jump.
Images	
Equipment	None or Aerofloor
Start	Start in a lunge position.
Action	Using your arms for momentum, drive upwards as high as possible and land in the same position in which you started. Repeat for the required number of reps.

Table 58

Exercise	Split squat with cycle.
Images	
Equipment	None or Aerofloor
Start	Start in a lunge position.
Action	Using your arms for momentum, drive upwards as high as possible while cycling your legs so you land in the lunge position but with your opposite leg furthest forward. Repeat for the required number of reps.

Table 59

Exercise	Pike jump.
Images	
Equipment	None or Aerofloor
Start	Start in an upright position.
Action	From an upright position jump up but only bending at the hips. You should try not to bend your knees, although hamstring and lower back flexibility will limit this. Reach forward to touch your toes at the highest point and land in the starting position.

Table 60

STANDING JUMPS

Exercise	Jump over barrier.
Images	
Equipment	Hurdle (This drill can use any size hurdle from 6in SAQ hurdle up to an Olympic hurdle)
Start	Stand in an upright position facing the hurdle with your feet a shoulder width apart.
Action	Squat down and, using a double arm drive, jump up and over the hurdle before landing in a bent knee position on the other side.

Table 61

Exercise	Lateral jump over barrier.
Images	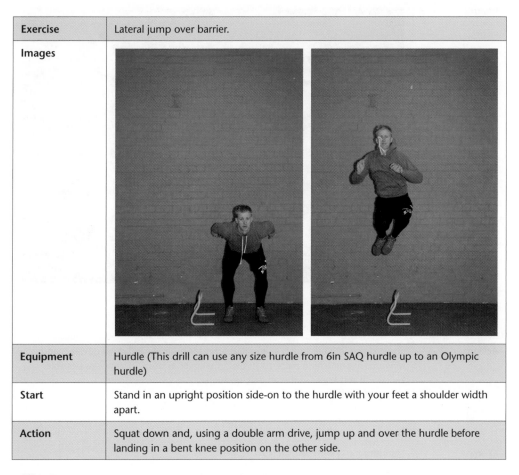
Equipment	Hurdle (This drill can use any size hurdle from 6in SAQ hurdle up to an Olympic hurdle)
Start	Stand in an upright position side-on to the hurdle with your feet a shoulder width apart.
Action	Squat down and, using a double arm drive, jump up and over the hurdle before landing in a bent knee position on the other side.

Table 62

Exercise	Long jump.
Images	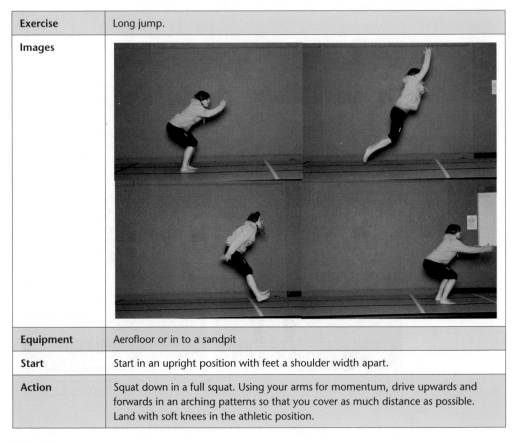
Equipment	Aerofloor or in to a sandpit
Start	Start in an upright position with feet a shoulder width apart.
Action	Squat down in a full squat. Using your arms for momentum, drive upwards and forwards in an arching patterns so that you cover as much distance as possible. Land with soft knees in the athletic position.

Table 63

Exercise	Standing jump with vertical reach.
Images	
Equipment	None
Start	Stand in an upright position with feet a shoulder width apart.
Action	Squat down and bring your hands behind you. Using a double arm drive, immediately drive upwards reaching as high as possible with both arms. Land in a bent leg position.

Table 64

Exercise	Single leg jump over barrier.
Images	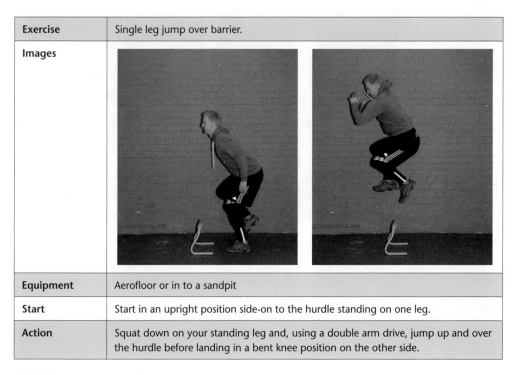
Equipment	Aerofloor or in to a sandpit
Start	Start in an upright position side-on to the hurdle standing on one leg.
Action	Squat down on your standing leg and, using a double arm drive, jump up and over the hurdle before landing in a bent knee position on the other side.

Table 65

Exercise	Alternating single leg lateral jump over barrier.
Images	
Equipment	Hurdle
Start	Stand on one leg next to the hurdle – the one furthest from the hurdle.
Action	Squat down on your standing leg and, using a double arm drive, jump up and over the hurdle before landing on the opposite leg in a bent knee position.

Table 66

Exercise	Single leg lateral jump over barrier.
Images	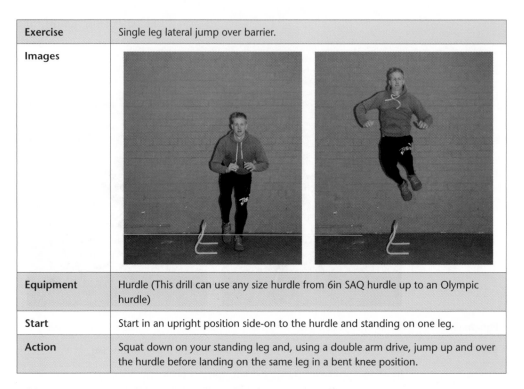
Equipment	Hurdle (This drill can use any size hurdle from 6in SAQ hurdle up to an Olympic hurdle)
Start	Start in an upright position side-on to the hurdle and standing on one leg.
Action	Squat down on your standing leg and, using a double arm drive, jump up and over the hurdle before landing on the same leg in a bent knee position.

Table 67

Exercise	Single leg long jump.
Images	
Equipment	Aerofloor or sandpit
Start	Stand in a vertical position on one leg.
Action	Squat down in a full squat. Using your arms for momentum, drive upwards and forwards in an arching pattern to cover as much distance as possible. Land on your jumping leg and regain your balance before standing on two feet to recover.

Table 68

Exercise	123 drill.
Images	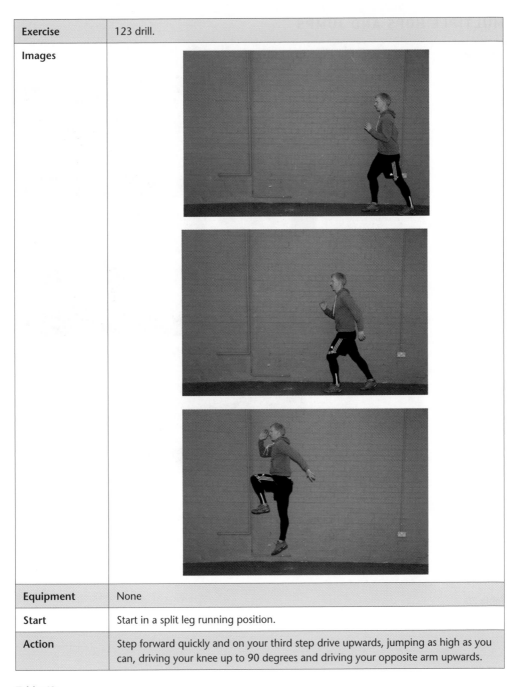
Equipment	None
Start	Start in a split leg running position.
Action	Step forward quickly and on your third step drive upwards, jumping as high as you can, driving your knee up to 90 degrees and driving your opposite arm upwards.

Table 69

MULTIPLE HOPS AND JUMPS

Exercise	Travelling squat jumps.
Images	
Equipment	None
Start	Start in a standing position with your feet a shoulder width apart and your hands behind your head.
Action	Squat down in a quarter squat, jumping immediately forwards. Repeat for the required number of reps or distance.

Table 70

Exercise	Multiple barrier jumps.
Images	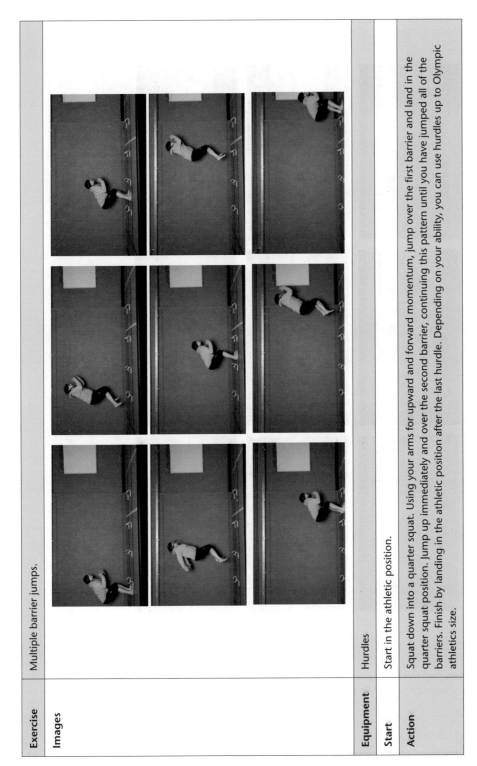
Equipment	Hurdles
Start	Start in the athletic position.
Action	Squat down into a quarter squat. Using your arms for upward and forward momentum, jump over the first barrier and land in the quarter squat position. Jump up immediately and over the second barrier, continuing this pattern until you have jumped all of the barriers. Finish by landing in the athletic position after the last hurdle. Depending on your ability, you can use hurdles up to Olympic athletics size.

Table 71

95

Exercise	Lateral barrier jumps.
Images	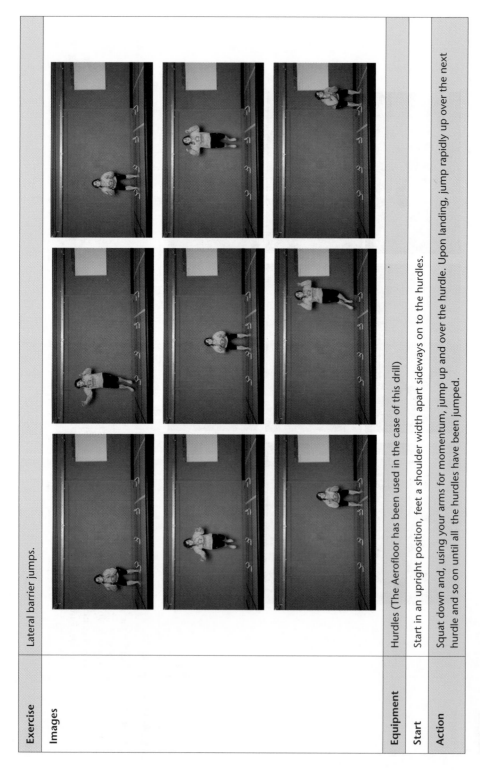
Equipment	Hurdles (The Aerofloor has been used in the case of this drill)
Start	Start in an upright position, feet a shoulder width apart sideways on to the hurdles.
Action	Squat down and, using your arms for momentum, jump up and over the hurdle. Upon landing, jump rapidly up over the next hurdle and so on until all the hurdles have been jumped.

Table 72

96

Exercise	Diagonal jumps.
Images	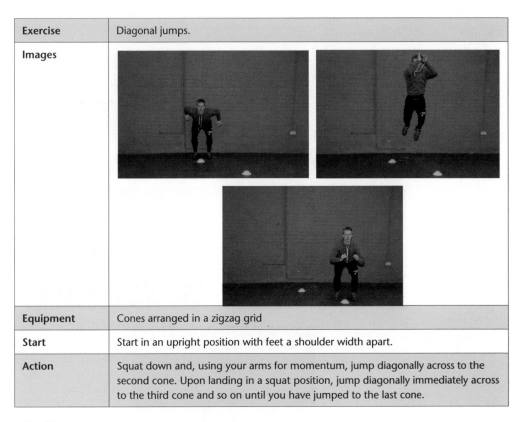
Equipment	Cones arranged in a zigzag grid
Start	Start in an upright position with feet a shoulder width apart.
Action	Squat down and, using your arms for momentum, jump diagonally across to the second cone. Upon landing in a squat position, jump diagonally immediately across to the third cone and so on until you have jumped to the last cone.

Table 73

Exercise	Zigzag jumps over cones.
Images	
Equipment	Cones or hurdles
Start	Start in a standing position with your feet a shoulder width apart.
Action	Squat down into a quarter squat and, using your arms for momentum, drive upwards jumping diagonally across the line of cones. Jump back immediately across the cones on landing, repeating this until you have reached the end of the cones or for the required number of reps.

Table 74

Exercise	Multiple barrier hops.
Images	
Equipment	Cones or small hurdles (The Aerofloor has been used in this drill)
Start	Stand in a vertical position on one leg.
Action	Squat down in a quarter squat. Using your arms for momentum, drive upwards jumping on to the box landing on your take-off leg. Stand up straight to finish before putting your resting foot down.

Table 75

Exercise	Lateral barrier hops.
Images	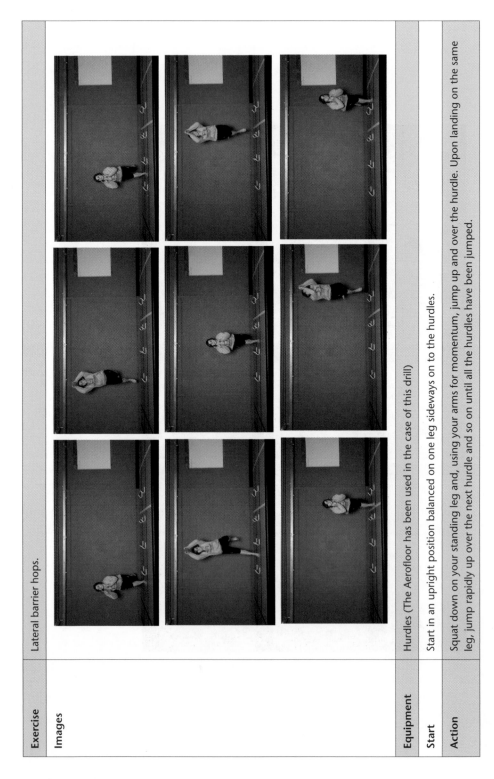
Equipment	Hurdles (The Aerofloor has been used in the case of this drill)
Start	Start in an upright position balanced on one leg sideways on to the hurdles.
Action	Squat down on your standing leg and, using your arms for momentum, jump up and over the hurdle. Upon landing on the same leg, jump rapidly up over the next hurdle and so on until all the hurdles have been jumped.

Table 76

Exercise	Diagonal hops.
Images	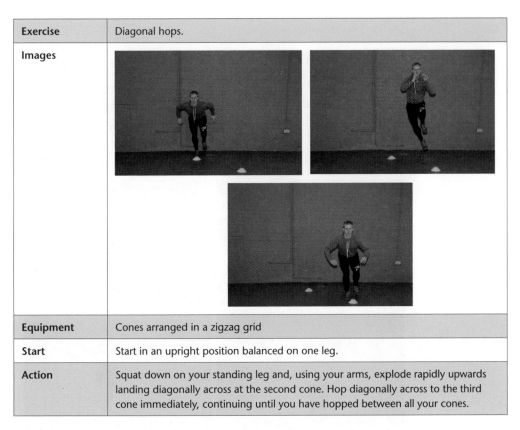
Equipment	Cones arranged in a zigzag grid
Start	Start in an upright position balanced on one leg.
Action	Squat down on your standing leg and, using your arms, explode rapidly upwards landing diagonally across at the second cone. Hop diagonally across to the third cone immediately, continuing until you have hopped between all your cones.

Table 77

Exercise	Single leg zigzag hops over cones.
Images	
Equipment	Cones or hurdles
Start	Stand in a vertical position on one leg.
Action	Squat down in a quarter squat on your standing leg. Using your arms for momentum, drive upwards jumping diagonally across the line of cones. Hop back immediately across the cones on landing, repeating this until you have reached the end of the cones or for the required number of reps.

Table 78

Exercise	Cone jumps with 180 degree turns.
Images	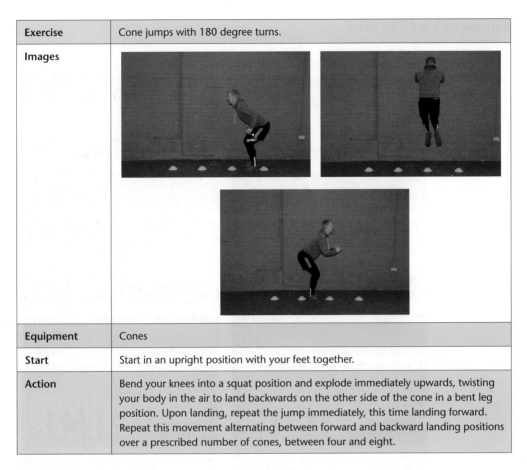
Equipment	Cones
Start	Start in an upright position with your feet together.
Action	Bend your knees into a squat position and explode immediately upwards, twisting your body in the air to land backwards on the other side of the cone in a bent leg position. Upon landing, repeat the jump immediately, this time landing forward. Repeat this movement alternating between forward and backward landing positions over a prescribed number of cones, between four and eight.

Table 79

BOUNDING EXERCISES

Exercise	Skipping.
Images	
Equipment	Aerofloor (or track)
Start	Start in an upright position.
Action	Skipping requires you to drive alternate legs and arms as you travel forward. Maintain a good knee and arm drive to propel yourself forward at speed. Ensure you cycle your legs quickly. Perform over 10–50m.

Table 80

Exercise	High skipping.
Images	
Equipment	Track (or Aerofloor)
Start	Start in an upright position.
Action	This drill requires you to skip with powerful vertical skips. Drive up as you skip so you achieve a maximum high point on each skip. Use alternate arm drive to increase your skipping height. Repeat for 10 to 50m.

Table 81

Exercise	Bounding with single arm action.
Images	
Equipment	Aerofloor (or track)
Start	Start in an upright position.
Action	Initiate momentum by driving one leg forward while driving your opposite arm forward. Hold your knee at 90 degrees for as long as possible before landing and performing the opposite leg and arm drive. You are trying to cover as much horizontal distance as possible in the shortest amount of 'bounds' as you travel along a required distance, usually 10–50m.

Table 82

Exercise	Bounding with Double Arm Action.
Images	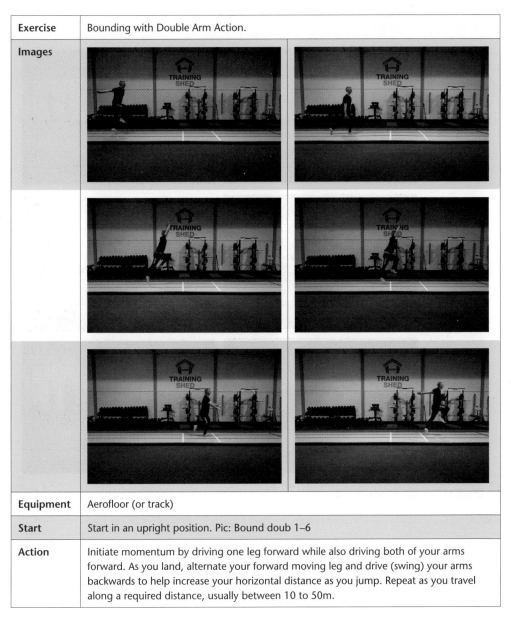
Equipment	Aerofloor (or track)
Start	Start in an upright position. Pic: Bound doub 1–6
Action	Initiate momentum by driving one leg forward while also driving both of your arms forward. As you land, alternate your forward moving leg and drive (swing) your arms backwards to help increase your horizontal distance as you jump. Repeat as you travel along a required distance, usually between 10 to 50m.

Table 83

Exercise	Single leg bound.
Images	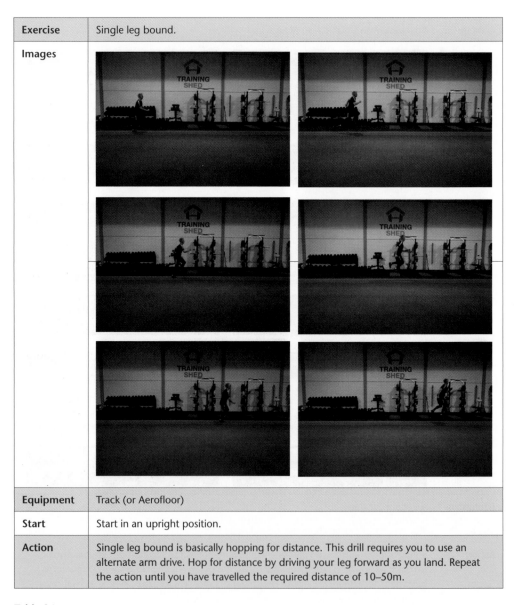
Equipment	Track (or Aerofloor)
Start	Start in an upright position.
Action	Single leg bound is basically hopping for distance. This drill requires you to use an alternate arm drive. Hop for distance by driving your leg forward as you land. Repeat the action until you have travelled the required distance of 10–50m.

Table 84

BOX DRILL EXERCISES

Exercise	Box landing.
Images	
Equipment	Soft plyometric boxes
Start	Stand in a vertical position on top of the plyometric box with your feet a shoulder width apart.
Action	Step forwards without jumping from the box and allow yourself to fall feet first towards the floor. Land in an athletic position – feet shoulder width apart in an upright position and your arms held out to the side in a bent arm relaxed position. Keep your head up and facing forward. The landing should be soft and the action of allowing your knees to bend will absorb your downward momentum upon landing. Stay relaxed upon landing but in control of your position. Your shoulders should be in alignment above your ankles so you are neither falling forwards nor backwards.

Table 85

Exercise	Two foot box jump.
Images	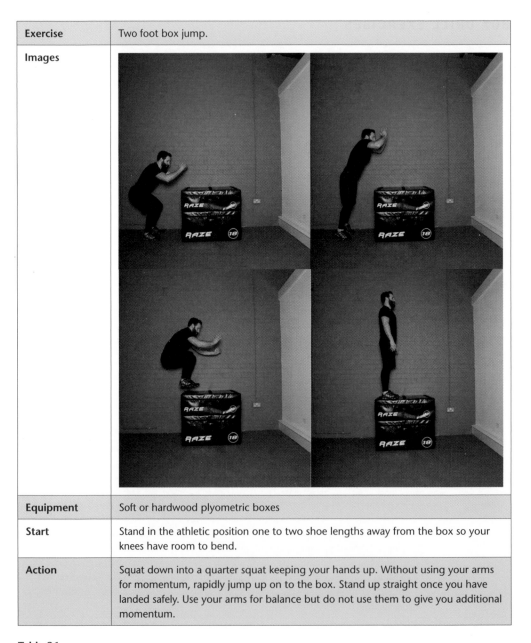
Equipment	Soft or hardwood plyometric boxes
Start	Stand in the athletic position one to two shoe lengths away from the box so your knees have room to bend.
Action	Squat down into a quarter squat keeping your hands up. Without using your arms for momentum, rapidly jump up on to the box. Stand up straight once you have landed safely. Use your arms for balance but do not use them to give you additional momentum.

Table 86

Exercise	Pyramid box jumps.
Images	
Equipment	Soft plyometric boxes of three different and increasing heights. Set the plyometric boxes in a line of three like a pyramid with enough room to land in between them safely.
Start	Stand with your feet shoulder width apart in an upright position.
Action	Squat down into a quarter squat and, using your arms for momentum, jump on to the lowest box, jumping off immediately and landing on the floor in the athletic position. Continue this process for the second and third boxes along the row.

Table 87

Exercise	Lateral box jump.
Images	
Equipment	Hardwood plyometric boxes
Start	Start in an upright position sideways on to the box.
Action	Start in the athletic position. Squat down and using your arms for upward momentum drive quickly upwards so you land on the box in the athletic position. As you land, jump immediately up laterally off the box and land on the opposite side of the box to where you started. You can perform this drill by jumping immediately back to where you started or for multiple reps back and forth across the box.

Table 88

Exercise	Single leg push off.
Images	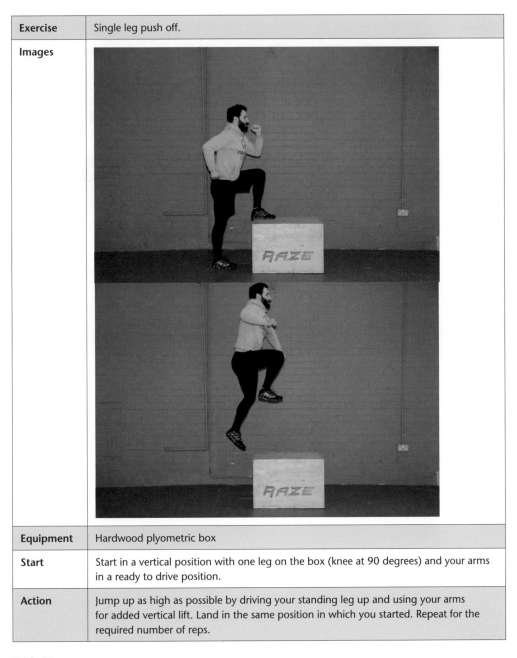
Equipment	Hardwood plyometric box
Start	Start in a vertical position with one leg on the box (knee at 90 degrees) and your arms in a ready to drive position.
Action	Jump up as high as possible by driving your standing leg up and using your arms for added vertical lift. Land in the same position in which you started. Repeat for the required number of reps.

Table 89

Exercise	Lateral leg push off
Images	
Equipment	Soft or hardwood plyometric boxes
Start	Stand in a vertical position with one leg on the plyo box and the other on the floor. Set your arm position for a split arm drive (pictured).
Action	Drive upwards with your leg positioned on the box while driving your standing leg simultaneously into a bent knee position. Use your arms to assist with your upward lift. Land softly in the starting position.

Table 90

Exercise	Alternate leg push off.
Images	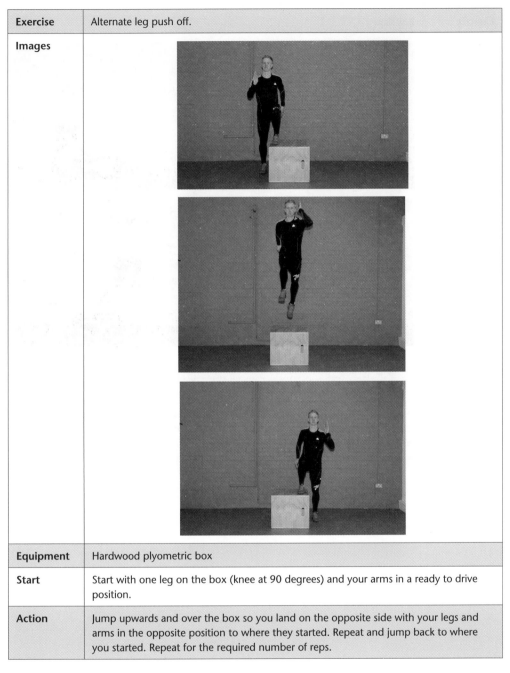
Equipment	Hardwood plyometric box
Start	Start with one leg on the box (knee at 90 degrees) and your arms in a ready to drive position.
Action	Jump upwards and over the box so you land on the opposite side with your legs and arms in the opposite position to where they started. Repeat and jump back to where you started. Repeat for the required number of reps.

Table 91

Exercise	Box skip.
Images	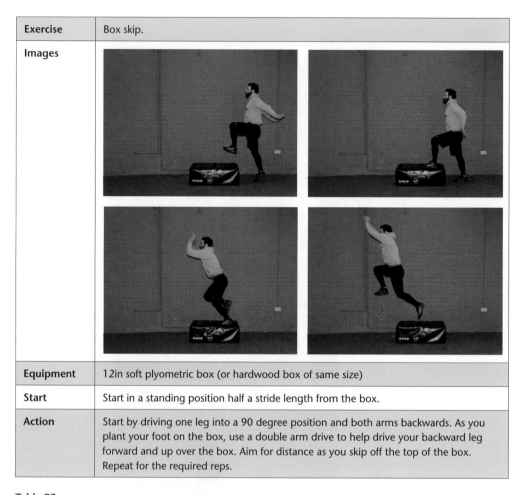
Equipment	12in soft plyometric box (or hardwood box of same size)
Start	Start in a standing position half a stride length from the box.
Action	Start by driving one leg into a 90 degree position and both arms backwards. As you plant your foot on the box, use a double arm drive to help drive your backward leg forward and up over the box. Aim for distance as you skip off the top of the box. Repeat for the required reps.

Table 92

Exercise	Box bound.
Images	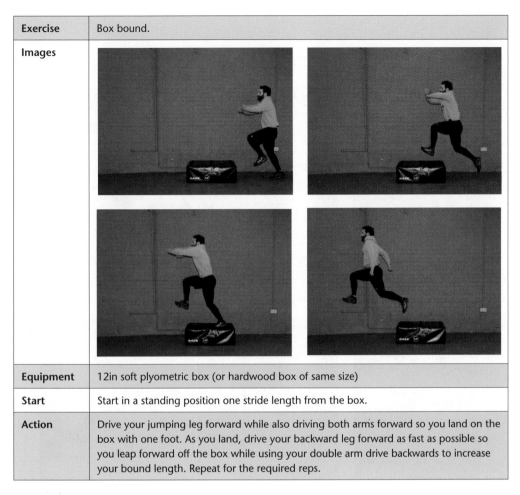
Equipment	12in soft plyometric box (or hardwood box of same size)
Start	Start in a standing position one stride length from the box.
Action	Drive your jumping leg forward while also driving both arms forward so you land on the box with one foot. As you land, drive your backward leg forward as fast as possible so you leap forward off the box while using your double arm drive backwards to increase your bound length. Repeat for the required reps.

Table 93

Exercise	Two foot multiple box jump.
Images	

Table 94

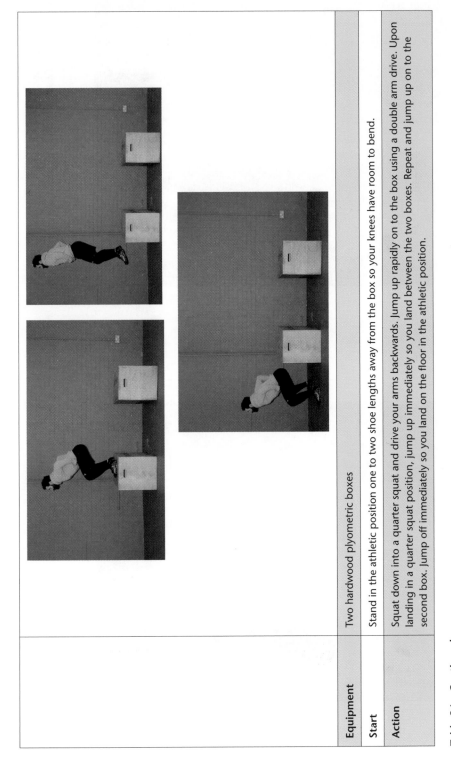

Equipment	Two hardwood plyometric boxes
Start	Stand in the athletic position one to two shoe lengths away from the box so your knees have room to bend.
Action	Squat down into a quarter squat and drive your arms backwards. Jump up rapidly on to the box using a double arm drive. Upon landing in a quarter squat position, jump up immediately so you land between the two boxes. Repeat and jump up on to the second box. Jump off immediately so you land on the floor in the athletic position.

Table 94 *Continued.*

Exercise	Two foot multiple box jump with hang.
Images	
Equipment	Two hardwood plyometric boxes
Action	As you land on the second box jump, jump up vertically quickly, reaching above your head and hanging in a vertical jump position for as long as possible before landing in an athletic position.

Table 95

Exercise	Two foot multiple box jump with tuck.
Images	
Equipment	Two hardwood plyometric boxes
Action	As you land on the second box jump, quickly jump up into a tuck position before landing in an athletic position.

Table 96

DEPTH JUMP EXERCISES

Exercise	Depth jump.
Images	
Equipment	Soft plyometric boxes
Start	Start in an upright position with your toes up against the edge of the box.
Action	Step forward from the box and drop to the floor, landing in an athletic position. Your arms should move to the backward position in a ready to drive up position. As soon as you land, and as quickly as possible, jump up rapidly as high as you can using your arms for momentum.

Table 97

Exercise	Depth leap.
Images	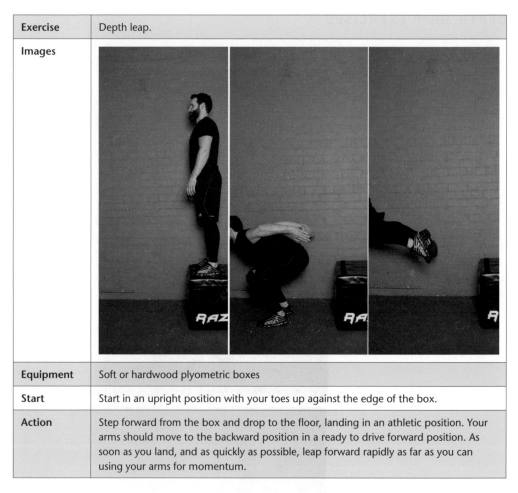
Equipment	Soft or hardwood plyometric boxes
Start	Start in an upright position with your toes up against the edge of the box.
Action	Step forward from the box and drop to the floor, landing in an athletic position. Your arms should move to the backward position in a ready to drive forward position. As soon as you land, and as quickly as possible, leap forward rapidly as far as you can using your arms for momentum.

Table 98

Exercise	Depth jump to box.
Images	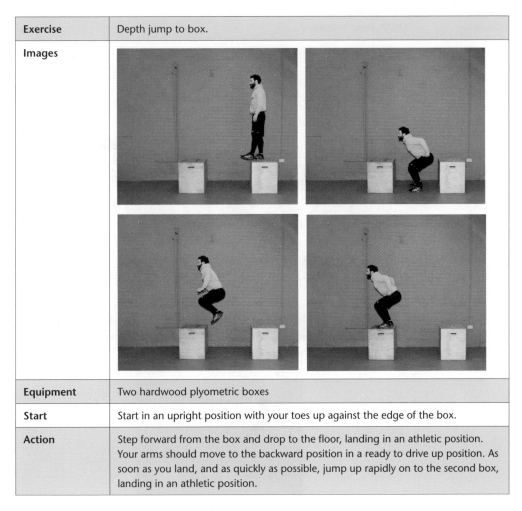
Equipment	Two hardwood plyometric boxes
Start	Start in an upright position with your toes up against the edge of the box.
Action	Step forward from the box and drop to the floor, landing in an athletic position. Your arms should move to the backward position in a ready to drive up position. As soon as you land, and as quickly as possible, jump up rapidly on to the second box, landing in an athletic position.

Table 99

Exercise	Depth Jump with leap.
Images	
Equipment	Two hardwood plyometric boxes
Start	Start in an upright position with your toes up against the edge of the box.
Action	Step forward from the box and drop to the floor, landing in an athletic position. Your arms should move to the backward position in a ready to drive up position. As soon as you land, and as quickly as possible, jump up rapidly on to the second box, landing in an athletic position. As you land on the box, leap off of it immediately while trying to achieve maximum distance in your leap.

Table 100

UPPER BODY PLYOS

Exercise	Vertical medicine ball throw.
Images	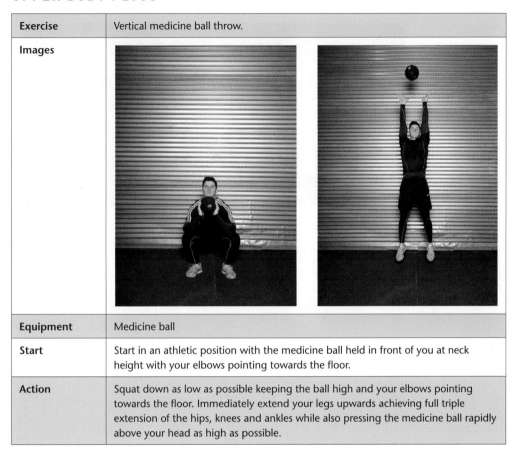
Equipment	Medicine ball
Start	Start in an athletic position with the medicine ball held in front of you at neck height with your elbows pointing towards the floor.
Action	Squat down as low as possible keeping the ball high and your elbows pointing towards the floor. Immediately extend your legs upwards achieving full triple extension of the hips, knees and ankles while also pressing the medicine ball rapidly above your head as high as possible.

Table 101

Exercise	Behind head throw.
Images	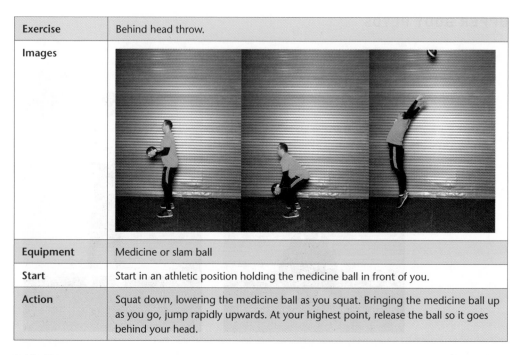
Equipment	Medicine or slam ball
Start	Start in an athletic position holding the medicine ball in front of you.
Action	Squat down, lowering the medicine ball as you squat. Bringing the medicine ball up as you go, jump rapidly upwards. At your highest point, release the ball so it goes behind your head.

Table 102

Exercise	Diagonal medicine ball throw.
Images	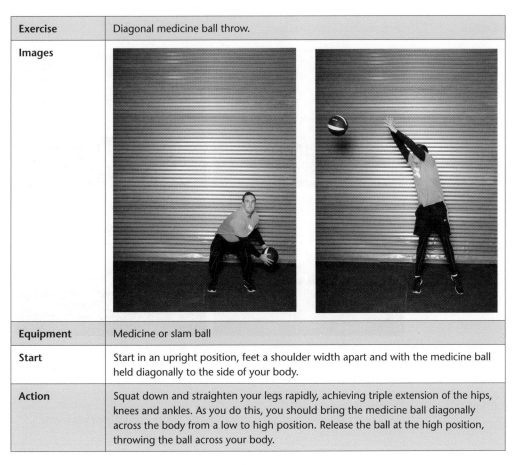
Equipment	Medicine or slam ball
Start	Start in an upright position, feet a shoulder width apart and with the medicine ball held diagonally to the side of your body.
Action	Squat down and straighten your legs rapidly, achieving triple extension of the hips, knees and ankles. As you do this, you should bring the medicine ball diagonally across the body from a low to high position. Release the ball at the high position, throwing the ball across your body.

Table 103

Exercise	Drop press-up from Airex pad.
Images	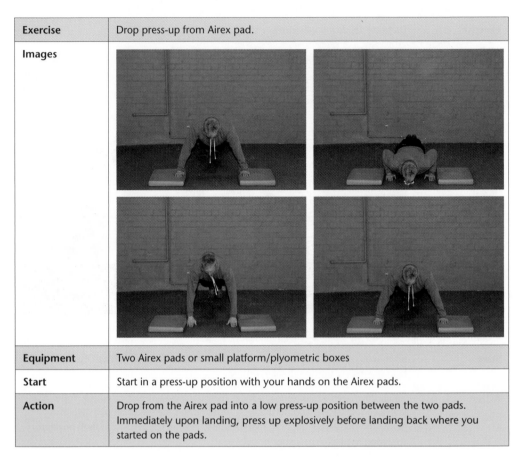
Equipment	Two Airex pads or small platform/plyometric boxes
Start	Start in a press-up position with your hands on the Airex pads.
Action	Drop from the Airex pad into a low press-up position between the two pads. Immediately upon landing, press up explosively before landing back where you started on the pads.

Table 104

Exercise	Power drop.
Images	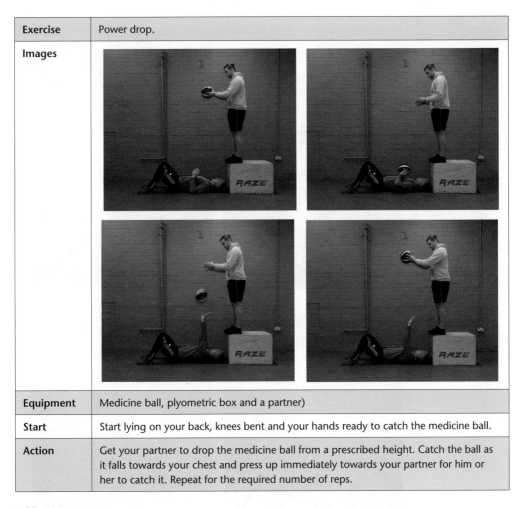
Equipment	Medicine ball, plyometric box and a partner)
Start	Start lying on your back, knees bent and your hands ready to catch the medicine ball.
Action	Get your partner to drop the medicine ball from a prescribed height. Catch the ball as it falls towards your chest and press up immediately towards your partner for him or her to catch it. Repeat for the required number of reps.

Table 105

Exercise	Medicine ball chest pass on knees with rebound press up.
Images	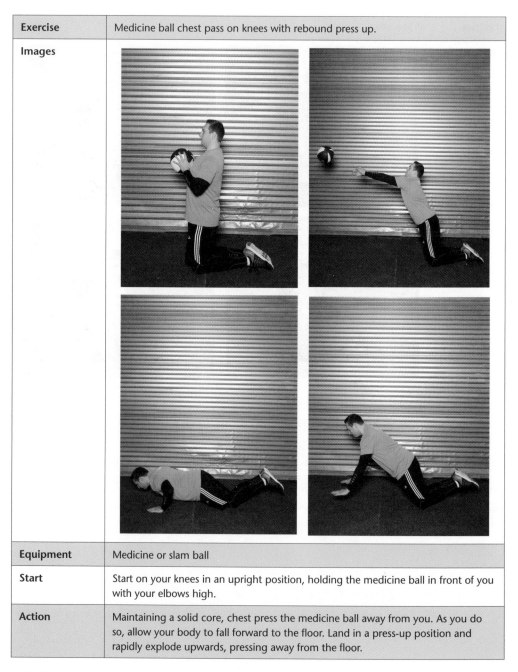
Equipment	Medicine or slam ball
Start	Start on your knees in an upright position, holding the medicine ball in front of you with your elbows high.
Action	Maintaining a solid core, chest press the medicine ball away from you. As you do so, allow your body to fall forward to the floor. Land in a press-up position and rapidly explode upwards, pressing away from the floor.

Table 106

Exercise	Split stance medicine ball throw.
Images	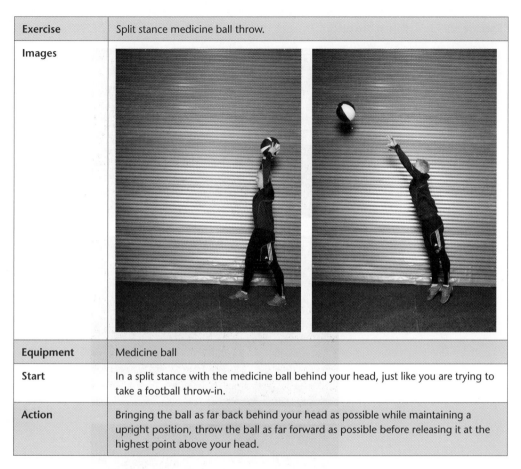
Equipment	Medicine ball
Start	In a split stance with the medicine ball behind your head, just like you are trying to take a football throw-in.
Action	Bringing the ball as far back behind your head as possible while maintaining an upright position, throw the ball as far forward as possible before releasing it at the highest point above your head.

Table 107

Exercise	Boxing bag push.
Images	
Equipment	Boxing bag
Start	Start in a split leg position with one hand flat against the boxing bag. Ensure the bag is level with your shoulders.
Action	Keeping a stable base, push the boxing bag rapidly forward as fast as possible.

Table 108

8 | PROGRAMMES

Any training programme you undertake should be specific to you. Before you begin you and/or your coach should undertake an athlete and sports specific needs analysis. This analysis should assess the physiological and biomechanical requirements of both the athlete and sport.

THE ATHLETE

Before embarking on your plyometric programme, you should have developed good motor control and functional strength based on the strength continuum mentioned in Chapter 4. All training programmes should start with the basics to ensure correct technique development for the athlete. Always start with simple drills of low intensity such as Jumps in Place, Standing Jumps and Footwork drills that will help the athlete to master important skills such as foot placement for both single-foot and double-foot take-offs and landings with sound biomechanics. Once they have demonstrated the required strength, stability and coordination the athlete can then move from general to specific or simple to complex drills as well as including sports specific drills.

Sports Specific

A practical approach to selecting the correct plyometric drills is to think about how you move in your sport and what physical action is taking place.

- Do I travel in a vertical or horizontal direction?
- Do I run?
- If I jump do I take off from one leg or two?
- Do I push with my arms or hit anything?

All of these questions are important to selecting the right drills and exercises for your sport. Table 109 shows a few examples of physical actions that occur in sports, which sport they occur and which type of plyometric drills might be useful. There are of course multiple answers for every action and column heading and this table is just to get you thinking.

Loading

The general consensus is that a beginner athlete should perform between 80 to 100 foot contacts of low-intensity drills such as Footwork Drills, Jumps in Place and Standing Jumps, with restricted volume medium intensity Multiple

Sport	Movement Example	Physical Action	Plyometric Drill Type	Drill Example
Any bipedal team sport	Movement around the court or pitch	Running	Bounding	Skipping
Athletics	Sprint starts	Acceleration	Jumps in Place	Two Foot Ankle Hops
Football	Running to support a break away	High velocity running	Bounding	Bounding with Single Arm Action
Volleyball	Jumping to block at the net	Jumping from two feet	Box Drills	Two Footed Box Jump
Basketball	Lay up	Jumping from one foot	Standing Jumps	123 Drill
Tennis	Forehand	Hitting	Upper Body Plyometrics	Diagonal MEDBall Throw
Martial Arts	Evading	Change of direction	Multiple Hops and Jumps – Footwork Drills	Diagonal Hops (and Any Footwork Drill)
Rugby	Scrummaging	Leg driving	Depth Jumps	Depth Jump
Kayaking/ Canoeing	Paddling	Twisting	Upper Body Plyometrics	Boxing Bag Push

Table 109   Plyometric drills for different sports.

Hops and Jump Drills once they are able to do so. An Intermediate athlete with some plyometrics experience should perform between 100 to 120 foot contacts using the drills previously learnt as a beginner but also moving to more moderate complexity drills such as Bounding and Box Drills. An advanced athlete should perform between 120 to 140 foot contacts of all the low and medium intensity drills as well as complex depth jumps drills.

The obvious point to make here is that every athlete and drill is different so you should look at both the competency of the athlete as well as the intensity of the drill. The more dynamic the drill, the more power is exerted performing movement, therefore fewer foot contacts should be observed. Also, an advanced athlete might be able to perform well beyond the recommended 100 to 120 foot contacts at low intensity drills, almost double the number, if their training readiness allows. As an athlete's training progresses, it is crucial to maintain quality and the number of foot contacts should be reduced, as optimum power and speed need to govern performance.

It is best to measure Bounding, Hops and Multiple Jumps in terms of sets and reps, distance covered and whether they are performed from a standing start or with a run-up. It is recommended to incorporate a maximum of 5–10 bounds per set into a session, with no more than 50–75 ground contacts. If a run-up

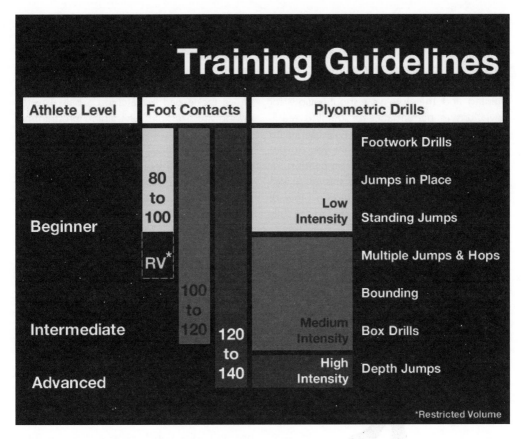

Table 110   Foot contact guidelines for plyometric training.

is used, the number of reps should be reduced. The main point here is to avoid fatiguing; rest between sets should be in the region of one or two minutes for any of the drills performed, although up to five minutes can be observed if performing maximal effort attempts. When it comes to depth jumps, between 15 to 30 seconds rest is recommended and some-times longer in cases of high intensity. Rest between drills and sets is as important as the work being performed. Recovery intervals will enable the stretch reflex mechanism to return to optimum readiness so that maximal power can be achieved.

Most athletes on a progressive plyometric training programme should adhere to a two or

Selecting depth jump box height

Research has shown that a Depth Jump Box height of 29 inches develops speed and up to 43 inches increases dynamic strength. Once you go beyond this height, the plyometric effect is reduced due to an increase in coupling time, i.e. the time it takes to land and take off again. The obvious rule is to increase Depth Jump box height only when the athlete is ready. Varying box heights lower than 29 inches has also been found to be effective in the development of plyometric training, indicating that it is the speed of *'coupling'* that should be an major factor in box height selection.

three times a week plyometric training plan. At least 24 hours rest between sessions, although 48 would be better. When starting a plyometric training programme, the forces and actions involved are very different to normal strength training and therefore you should allow for deviations in performance or training readiness as the body adapts to this type of training modality. You should ensure that you do not perform plyometrics before competition or an important calendar event as this could also affect your performance. A standard taper of seven to twelve days will ensure you are fully prepared for competition.

This book gives you a flavour of the plyometric exercises available to a coach or athlete. As you become more experienced, you can tailor some these exercises to your sport by adding a sport-specific movement or skill such as driving into a tackle pad or catching a ball. The following are examples of training programmes that I have used with great success. Remember that all programmes you undertake should be specific to the athlete and not simply a replication of somebody else's training. Therefore use the following sample programmes as a guide to help you plan your way to improved speed and power in your sport.

BASKETBALL/NETBALL

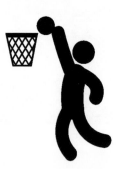

Basketball and netball are court sports that require exceptional agility and speed of movement. The need to jump, whether performing a lay-up or block, is also key to performance in basketball, with both sports requiring the ability to jump vertically from a static position. This programme develops multi-directional speed and agility, jump height and passing power.

BEGINNER			
Exercise/Drill	**Drill Type**	**Reps**	**Sets**
Hexagon grid drill	Footwork drill		3–6
Two foot ankle hop		10	2
Star jump	Jumps in place	6	2
Rocket jump		6	2
123 drill	Standing jumps	6	2 (EL)
Standing vertical jump with reach		6	2
		Total foot contacts 80	
Split stance overhead med ball throw	Upper body plyos	8	2

Table 111

FOOTWORK DRILLS

Exercise	Four Square (each square is 60cm)
Image	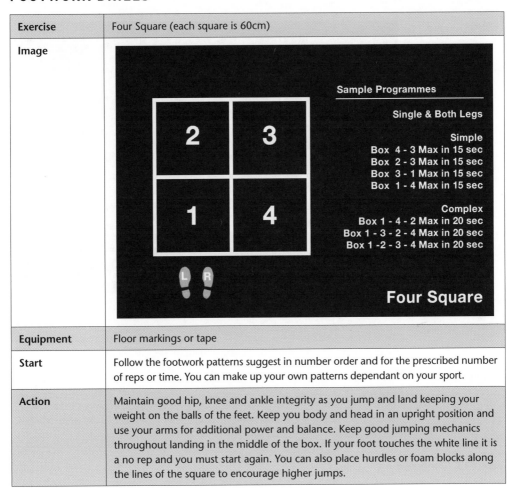
Equipment	Floor markings or tape
Start	Follow the footwork patterns suggest in number order and for the prescribed number of reps or time. You can make up your own patterns dependant on your sport.
Action	Maintain good hip, knee and ankle integrity as you jump and land keeping your weight on the balls of the feet. Keep you body and head in an upright position and use your arms for additional power and balance. Keep good jumping mechanics throughout landing in the middle of the box. If your foot touches the white line it is a no rep and you must start again. You can also place hurdles or foam blocks along the lines of the square to encourage higher jumps.

Table 112

Exercise	Nine Square (each square is 40cm)
Image	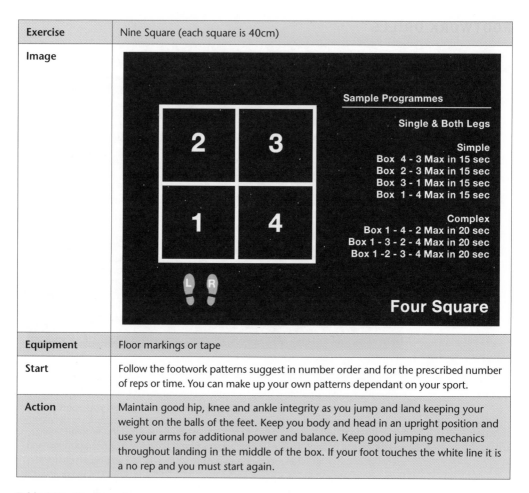
Equipment	Floor markings or tape
Start	Follow the footwork patterns suggest in number order and for the prescribed number of reps or time. You can make up your own patterns dependant on your sport.
Action	Maintain good hip, knee and ankle integrity as you jump and land keeping your weight on the balls of the feet. Keep you body and head in an upright position and use your arms for additional power and balance. Keep good jumping mechanics throughout landing in the middle of the box. If your foot touches the white line it is a no rep and you must start again.

Table 112   Continued.

INTERMEDIATE			
Exercise/Drill	**Drill Type**	**Reps**	**Sets**
Four square drill	Footwork drill		3–6
Two foot ankle twist hop	Jumps in place	10	2
Split squat with cycle		6	2
Lateral barrier jump		6	2 (ES)
Zigzag jump over cones	Multiple hops and jumps	8	3
Cone jump with 180 degree turn		6	2
Two footed box jump with hang	Box drills	6	2
Alternate leg push off		8	2
		Total foot contacts 120	
Chest pass throw on knees with rebound press	Upper body plyos	8	3

Table 113

ADVANCED			
Exercise/Drill	**Drill Type**	**Reps**	**Sets**
Nine square drill	Footwork drill		3–6
Side to side ankle hop	Jumps in place	6	2 (EL)
Split squat with cycle		6	2
Alternating lateral jump over barrier	Standing jumps	10	2
Lateral barrier hop	Multiple hops and jumps	6	2 (EL)
Zigzag jump over cones		6	2
High skipping	Bounding	8	2
Two footed box with tuck jump	Box drills	4	2
Depth jump to box with leap	Depth jump	4	3
		Total foot contacts 138	
Power drop	Upper body plyos	10	2

Table 114

CYCLING

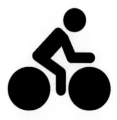

Although cycling is a seated sport, the positive gains that can be made from plyometrics are essential for performance. Cycling requires immense single leg strength as you transfer power to your wheels through every pedal stroke. The time that you obviously require more power is when you sprint and bike uphill. Starting with simple double leg drills and progressing through to single leg vertical drills is a great way to improve your cycling performance.

BEGINNER			
Exercise/Drill	Drill Type	Reps	Sets
Hexagon grid drill	Footwork drill		3–6
Two foot ankle hop	Jumps in place	10	2
Pike jump		6	2
Squat jump		6	2
123 drill	Standing jumps	6	2
Single leg jump over barrier		6	2 (EL)
		Total foot contacts 80	
Diagonal med ball throw	Upper body plyos	6	2

Table 115

INTERMEDIATE			
Exercise/Drill	Drill Type	Reps	Sets
Four square drill	Footwork drill		3–6
Two foot ankle hop	Jumps in place	10	3
Split squat jump		8	2
Travelling squat jump	Multiple hops and jumps	6	2
Bounding with double arm action	Bounding	10	2
Two footed box jump	Box drills	6	2
Single leg push off		6	2 (EL)
		Total foot contacts 114	
Diagonal med ball throw	Upper body plyos	8	4

Table 116

ADVANCED			
Exercise/Drill	Drill Type	Reps	Sets
Nine square drill	Footwork drill		3–6
Pike jump	Jumps in place	6	3
Slit squat jumps with cycle		8	2
Single leg bound	Bounding	10	2 (EL)
Skipping (fast)		10	2
Alternate leg push off	Box drills	6	2 (EL)
Depth jump	Depth jump	6	3
Total foot contacts 136			
Diagonal med ball throw	Upper body plyos	8	6

Table 117

FOOTBALL

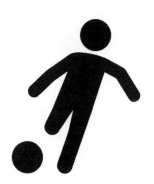

Football requires great acceleration, speed and agility. Footballers jump to head balls so both horizontal and vertical plyometrics need to be trained. Starting with simple two foot drills, this programme progresses through to single leg complex drills that will increase multidirectional speed. The need for good core control during twisting and turning movements is also necessary.

BEGINNER			
Exercise/Drill	Drill Type	Reps	Sets
Hexagon grid drill	Footwork drill		3–6
Foot ankle twist hop	Jumps in place	10	2
Box landing		6	2
Rocket jump		6	2
Jump over barrier	Standing jumps	6	2
Single leg long jump		8	3
Total foot contacts 80			
Behind head throw	Upper body plyos	6	2

Table 118

INTERMEDIATE			
Exercise/Drill	**Drill Type**	**Reps**	**Sets**
Four square drill	Footwork drill		3–6
Alternating single lateral leg jump over barrier	Standing jumps	6	3
Lateral barrier hop	Multiple hops and jumps	6	3
Diagonal hop		6	2
Zigzag jump over cones		10	3
Bounding with single arm action	Bounding	10	3
Two footed box jump with hang box drill		6	2
		Total foot contacts 120	
Split stance med ball throw	Upper body plyos	6	2

Table 119

ADVANCED			
Exercise/Drill	**Drill Type**	**Reps**	**Sets**
Nine square drill	Footwork drill		3–6
Single foot side to side ankle hop	Jumps in place	6	2 (EL)
Single leg long jump	Standing jumps	6	3 (EL)
Single leg zigzag hop over cones	Multiple hops & jumps	6	2
Skipping (fast)	Bounding	10	3
Lateral leg push off	Box drills	8	2
Depth jump	Depth jump	5	2
		Total foot contacts 140	
Diagonal med ball throw	Upper body plyos	6	2 (ES)

Table 120

MARTIAL ARTS

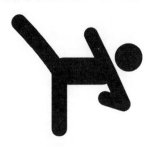

Martial arts require full body power, from evading an opponent, to punching, kicking, jumping, blocking and throwing. Leg power and upper body power are essential. This programme will develop full body speed and agility in equal measures.

BEGINNER			
Exercise/Drill	**Drill Type**	**Reps**	**Sets**
Hexagon grid drill	Footwork drill		3–6
Two foot ankle hop	Jumps in place	10	2
Star jump		6	2
Tuck jump knees up		6	2
Lateral jump over barrier	Standing jumps	6	2 (EL)
Long jump		6	2
		Total foot contacts 80	
Boxing bag push	Upper body plyos	6	2
Diagonal med ball throw		6	2 (ES)

Table 121

INTERMEDIATE			
Exercise/Drill	**Drill Type**	**Reps**	**Sets**
Four square drill	Footwork drill		3–6
Two foot ankle twist hop	Jumps in place	10	2
Tuck jump with butt kick		6	2
Diagonal hop	Multiple hops and jumps	6	2 (EL)
Zigzag jump over cones		8	2
Cone jump with 180 degree turn		6	2
Single leg box jump	Box drills	6	2
Pyramid box jump	Box drills	4	2
		Total foot contacts 120	
Vertical med ball throw with squat	Upper body plyos	6	2
Chest pass throw on knees with rebound press		6	2
Boxing bag push		6	2 (ES)

Table 122

ADVANCED			
Exercise/Drill	**Drill Type**	**Reps**	**Sets**
Nine square drill	Footwork drill		3–6
Side to side ankle hop	Jumps in place	6	2 (EL)
Split squat with cycle		8	2
Alternating lateral jump over barrier	Standing jumps	10	2
Multiple barrier hop	Multiple hops and jumps	8	2 (EL)
Zigzag jump over cones		6	2
Two footed box with tuck jump	Box drills	5	2
Depth leap	Depth jump	6	2
		Total foot contacts 138	
Power drop	Upper body plyos	10	2
Boxing bag push		10	2 (ES)
Drop press from Airex pad		6	2

Table 123

RACQUET SPORTS

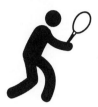

Racquet sports require great single leg agility and power as you lunge, jump and change direction rapidly to get into a strong hitting position. Single leg drills are essential to develop this neuromuscular coordination, whilst lateral and diagonal drills will mimic movements observed on the court.

BEGINNER			
Exercise/Drill	Drill Type	Reps	Sets
Hexagon grid drill	Footwork drill		3–6
Two foot ankle twist hop		10	2
Star jump	Jumps in place	6	2
Split squat jump		6	2
Lateral jump over barrier	Standing jumps	6	2 (EL)
Standing vertical jump with reach		6	2
		Total foot contacts 80	
Boxing bag push	Upper body plyos	6	2

Table 124

INTERMEDIATE			
Exercise/Drill	Drill Type	Reps	Sets
Four square drill	Footwork drill		3–6
Alternating single lateral leg jump over barrier	Standing jumps	8	3
Diagonal hop		6	2 (EL)
Single leg zigzag jump over cones	Multiple hops and jumps	8	2
Cone jump with 180 degree turn		8	3
Single leg box jump	Box drills	6	2
		Total foot contacts 118	
Diagonal med ball throw	Upper body plyos	6	2

Table 125

ADVANCED			
Exercise/Drill	**Drill Type**	**Reps**	**Sets**
Nine square drill	Footwork drill		3–6
Side to side ankle hop	Jumps in place	6	2 (EL)
Split squat with cycle		6	2
Single lateral leg jump over barrier	Standing jumps	6	2 (EL)
Single leg zigzag hop over cones	Multiple hops and jumps	8	3
Zigzag jump over cones		6	2
Single leg push off	Box drills	5	2
Depth jump to box with leap	Depth jump	5	2
		Total foot contacts 140	
Power drop	Upper body plyos	10	2

Table 126

RUGBY

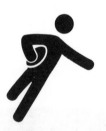

The rugby programme is designed to develop all body power. Rugby is a demanding game involving multi-direction movements involving both upper and lower body power. Sound mechanics must be observed before moving through the stages, where change of direction plyometrics become important to developing an agile and powerful player.

BEGINNER			
Exercise/Drill	**Drill Type**	**Reps**	**Sets**
Hexagon grid drill	Footwork drill		3–6
Two foot ankle hop	Jumps in place	10	2
Box landing		6	2
Squat jump		6	2
Single leg lateral jump over barrier	Standing jumps	6	2
Standing vertical jump with reach		8	3
		Total foot contacts 80	

Table 127

Boxing bag push	Upper body plyos	6	3
Diagonal med ball throw		6	3

Table 127   *Continued.*

INTERMEDIATE			
Exercise/Drill	**Drill Type**	**Reps**	**Sets**
Four square drill	Footwork drill		3–6
Alternate single lateral leg jump over barrier	Standing jumps	6	3
Travelling squat jump	Multiple hops and jumps	6	2
Skipping	Bounding	10	3
Bounding with single arm action		10	3
Pyramid box jump	Box drills	5	2
		Total foot contacts 120	
Power drop	Upper body plyos	6	3
Split stance overhead med ball throw		6	3

Table 128

ADVANCED			
Exercise/Drill	**Drill Type**	**Reps**	**Sets**
Nine square drill	Footwork drill		3–6
Pike jump	Jumps in place	6	3
Single leg long jump	Standing jumps	6	3 (EL)
Single leg zigzag hop over cones	Multiple hops & jumps	8	2
Skipping (fast)	Bounding	10	4
Two footed box jump with tuck jump	Box jumps	6	1
Depth jump to box	Depth jump	6	2
		Total foot contacts 140	
Drop press-up from Airex pad	Upper body plyos	6	3
Chest pass throw on knees with rebound press-up		6	3

Table 129

RUNNING

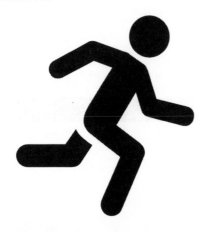

Most runners just run – which is crazy when you understand one simple fact. If you're stronger, you will be faster. There is the obvious caveat that you must train to be running strong, not just hitting the weights. So developing your strength using the continuum in Chapter 4 is the best place to start. Developing good functional running strength will make you less prone to injury too, which is always a bonus when you are training for a long distance run and need to get the miles in. The next step is to develop good running speed or power through the use of single leg and horizontal or linear plyometrics. Bounding drills are especially good for developing running speed.

BEGINNER			
Exercise/Drill	**Drill Type**	**Reps**	**Sets**
Hexagon grid drill	Footwork drill		3–6
Two foot ankle hop	Jumps in place	10	2
Pike jump		6	2
Split squat jump		6	2
Tick jump with butt kick		6	2
Single leg long jump	Standing jumps	6	2
		Total foot contacts 80	
Diagonal med ball throw	Upper body plyos	6	2

Table 130

INTERMEDIATE			
Exercise/Drill	**Drill Type**	**Reps**	**Sets**
Four square drill	Footwork drill		3–6
Split squat jump with cycle	Jumps in place	6	2
Multiple barrier jump	Multiple hops and jumps	6	2
Skipping	Bounding	10	3
Bounding with single arm action		10	4

Table 131

Single leg bound		6	2
	Total foot contacts 118		
Diagonal med ball throw	Upper body plyos	8	4

Table 131 *Continued.*

ADVANCED			
Exercise/Drill	**Drill Type**	**Reps**	**Sets**
Nine square drill	Footwork drill		3–6
Pike jump	Jumps in place	6	2
Multiple barrier hop	Multiple hops and jumps	8	2
Skipping (fast)	Bounding	10	2
Bounding with single arm action		10	4
Single leg bound		10	2 (EL)
Depth jump to box		6	2
	Total foot contacts 140		
Diagonal med ball throw	Upper body plyos	8	6

Table 132

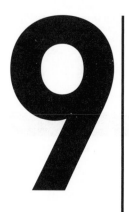

PERFORMANCE TESTING

Testing is always considered to be a serious subject but this should not be the case. You may have heard this before but I truly believe testing is training and training is testing and it should therefore form part of any training schedule or periodized plan. From an athletic standpoint, you should always use performance tests as they are a great way to collect meaningful information that can help in many ways. This information enables both athletes and coaches to understand where they currently are in their performance and enables the correct developmental programming to be administered in order to increase their performance.

The typical plyometric performance test that usually springs to the mind of any athlete or coach is a two-legged jump, either vertical or horizontal. These tests can be either static without a preload or with a preload countermovement where the athlete squats down pre-jump to elicit the stretch-shortening cycle. Most of us have performed or coached one of these jump tests at some point, whether it be at school or during a training programme. However, there are many other ways that you can test your explosive plyometric power and athletic development.

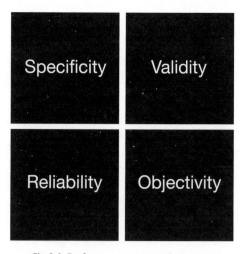

Fig 9.1 Performance test requirements.

HOW TO SELECT THE CORRECT TEST

First you should ask yourself: Why am I testing? What is it that I am trying to test? When selecting a performance test you should always consider these two questions as testing with no real purpose is neither useful nor worthwhile. Once you have answered these two questions you must then look to select or design a specific test that assesses exactly what it is you are trying to find out. All too often athletes and coaches go through a complicated battery of testing that is both unnecessary for their chosen sport or simply does not give them purposeful information.

First and foremost, you should only ever aim to measure one factor in your tests and this way you will get a true and accurate result. All performance tests must be objective rather than subjective, that is they must give you a specified numerical value on a performance movement rather than a coach's opinion of whether that 'looked good or not'. The test must have a standardized procedure, including a prescribed warm-up that every athlete must follow exactly. Pre-testing factors such as no caffeine, meals eaten, time of day that you are testing and so on (see list below) are all factors that must be taken into consideration by any athlete or coach. The assessor must try to limit as many influencing factors as possible. This ensures the test is easily replicated and will reproduce a consistent process and result, irrespective of who is testing.

FACTORS AFFECTING TEST RELIABILITY

Use this checklist to reduce as many variables as possible when designing your test procedure.

- The ambient temperature, noise level and humidity
- The amount of sleep the athlete had prior to testing
- The athlete's emotional state
- Medication the athlete may be taking
- The time of day you are testing
- The athlete's caffeine intake
- The time since the athlete's last meal
- The test environment – surface (track, grass, road, gym)
- The athlete's prior test knowledge/experience
- Accuracy of measurements (times, distances and so on)

- Is the athlete actually applying maximum effort in maximal tests?
- Inappropriate warm-up
- The personality, knowledge and skill of the tester
- Athlete's clothing/shoes
- Surface on which the test is conducted
- Environmental conditions – wind, rain and so on.

WHAT TO DO WITH THE RESULTS

Once you have performed the test and have some objective data to evaluate, you must use this information to help you implement some valid decisions. This process should always involve the athlete as it will empower both of your roles within the athlete-coach relationship. Results from tests can give you a whole host of information. Most notably, and more often than not, they are used to predict future performance as the ability to achieve a specific test result will have a relationship with your performance levels in your chosen sport. Test results can help to place athletes in the correct training groups so they are not overreaching or over-training at levels that are not sustainable for continued improvement, and can act as a very good motivating tool for the athlete. All athletes and coaches are competitive by nature and, as well as satisfying the demand for competition for the athlete, testing also provides feedback to the coach on how well their training programme has gone. In more complex testing batteries, where multiple tests are used, testing can also help to highlight an area of weakness in an athlete's fitness profile.

PLYOMETRIC PERFORMANCE TESTS

The following tests are typical of plyometric performance evaluations and will enable you to test and score yourself with maximal efforts. There should be complete rest between each jump or throw performance of between three and five minutes. All test target scores are from my personal experience and should be used as guidelines and not ultimate performance reflectors. These tests are indicators of potential sports performance and are not exclusive in predicting champions. When analyzing tests, you should always use comparative previous athlete results and your own sports-specific athlete comparisons rather than generalized tables of standards.

Jump Tests

As mentioned previously, these are generally considered to be the 'plyometric tests' of

choice. They are often used in school settings as they are easily administered with little equipment and are safe for almost every athlete to perform. Jump tests can take a variety of forms, single leg, double leg, vertical, horizontal, single jumps and multiple jumps. The following are just a few of the protocols you can use to assess jump height and distance.

Static Vertical Jump (SVJ)

Also known as the Sargent Jump Test, the Static Vertical Jump was developed by Dr Dudley Allen Sargent in 1921 and is used to measure two-legged vertical jump power.

Equipment
• Wall • Tape measure • Stepladder • Chalk • Assistant
Procedure
1. The athlete follows a pre-described warm-up protocol. 2. The athlete chalks the middle finger of the hand that is closest to the wall (athlete is standing sideways). 3. The athlete reaches as high as is physically possible without leaning or lifting his or her feet. 4. The athlete should step 12–15cm sideways away from the wall to allow room to jump and reach. 5. The athlete squats down slowly into a quarter or full squat position (keep this start position consistent). 6. The athlete then jumps as high as possible, swinging his or her arms up and reaching as high as possible, placing a mark on the wall with a chalked finger. 7. Repeat the test three times. 8. The assistant measures the distance between the standing chalk mark and the highest placed chalk mark.

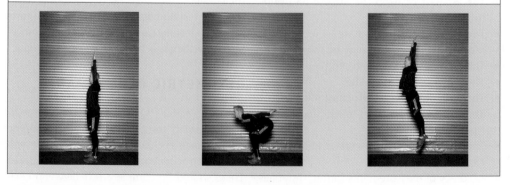

Table 133   Target scores for SVJ.

Target scores

	Female		Male	
	Junior	**Adult**	**Junior**	**Adult**
Excellent	52.5cm	55cm	68cm	70cm
Good	40–52.5cm	42.5–55cm	55–68cm	65–70cm
Average	30–40cm	32.5–42.5cm	42.5–55cm	52.5–65cm
More training required	<30cm	<32.5cm	<42.5cm	<52.5cm

Table 133 *Continued.*

Counter Movement Jump (CMJ)

This is probably one of the most used plyometric tests as it assesses the stretch-shortening cycle and its effect on power pro-duction during vertical jumps. It is similar in nature to that of the static or Sargant jump but with a pre-movement (loading) and rapid unloading squat movement.

Equipment
• Wall • Tape measure • Stepladder • Chalk • Assistant
Procedure
1. The athlete follows a pre-described warm-up protocol. 2. The athlete chalks the middle finger of the hand that is closest to the wall (athlete is standing sideways). 3. The athlete reaches as high as is physically possible without leaning or lifting his or her feet. 4. The athlete should step 12 to 15cm sideways away from the wall to allow room to jump and reach. 5. The athlete starts with hands above the head and squats down quickly into a full squat position, swinging his or her arms down and backwards. 6. The athlete then jumps rapidly (without pause) as high as possible, swinging his or her arms up and reaching as high as possible placing a mark on the wall with a chalked finger. 7. Repeat the test three times. 8. The assistant measures the distance between the standing chalk mark and the highest placed chalk mark.

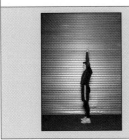 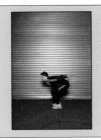 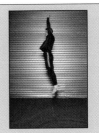

Running Vertical Jump (RVJ)

This plyometric test assesses power under higher loads and stress due to the three to five step movement pattern prior to the vertical jump. This test can be performed with a double or single leg take-off.

Equipment
• Vertec • Assistant

Procedure
1. The athlete follows a pre-described warm-up protocol. 2. The athlete stands underneath the Vertec reaching up as high as possible without leaning or lifting his or her feet. 3. The athlete then steps back three to five steps (or a specified amount) away from the Vertec. 4. The athlete then approaches the Vertec at speed aiming to execute the high point of the jump at the Vertec. 5. Repeat the test three times. 6. The assistant measures the height of the jump.

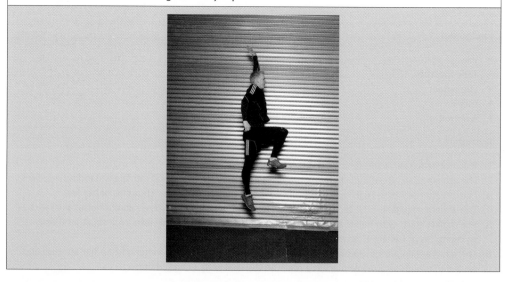

Target scores

	Female	Male
Excellent	60cm	70cm
Good	51–60cm	61–70cm
Average	31–40cm	41–50cm
More training required	<31cm	<41cm

Table 134 Target scores for RVJ.

Standing Broad Jump

Also known as the Long Jump Test, this test assesses horizontal jump performance.

Equipment
• Long jump pit (not essential but preferred) • Tape measure • Assistant

Procedure
1. The athlete follows a pre-described warm-up protocol. 2. The athlete stands with his or her feet against a marked starting line or edge of the long jump pit. 3. The athlete squats and, using his or her arms, jumps forward as far as possible, landing with both feet. 4. The assistant measures the back foot's distance from the starting mark. 5. Repeat the test three times. 6. The assistant uses the longest of the three jumps as the final result.

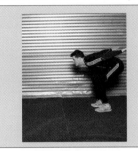 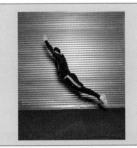 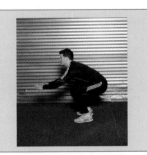

Target scores

	Female	Male
Excellent	>200cm	>250cm
Very good	191–200cm	241–250cm
Good	181–190cm	231–241cm
Average	171–181cm	221–231cm
More training required	<171cm	<221cm

Table 135   Target scores for standing broad jump.

Interesting Fact

The Standing Long Jump Test world record is held by Norwegian Arne Tvervaag from Ringerike FIK Sportclub, who jumped 3.71m in Noresund on 11 November 1968.

UPPER BODY PLYOMETRIC TESTS

Medicine Ball Chest Throw

This test is a great measurement of upper body power and easily administered. You should always use the same weight medicine ball, either a 4kg, 5kg or 6kg.

Equipment
• Medicine Ball • Tape measure • Assistant

Procedure
1. The athlete follows a pre-described warm-up protocol. 2. The athlete stands in an athletic position, holding the medicine ball at chest height and hands placed on either side of the medicine ball with fingers backwards to the chest. 3. The athlete chest throws the medicine ball as far as possible. 4. Repeat the test three times. 5. The assistant uses the longest of the three throws as the final result.

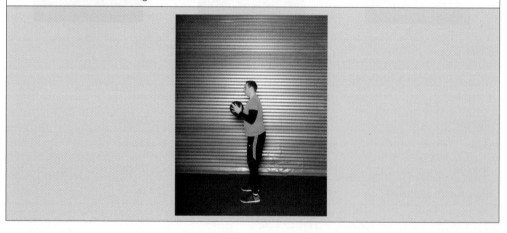

Target scores

Any test result shorter than 9m would suggest further upper body strength training is required or a lighter medicine ball should be used.

Overhead Forward Medicine Ball Throw

This test is a great measurement of upper body and explosive power. The movement is similar to that of a football throw-in. You should always use the same weight medicine ball, either a 2kg or 5kg depending in the age and experience of the person being tested. This test can be done from a feet side-by-side or one-foot-in-front-of-the-other position.

Equipment
• Medicine ball • Tape measure • Assistant

Procedure
1. The athlete follows a pre-described warm-up protocol. 2. The athlete stands in an athletic position, holding the medicine ball above their head with his or her hands on the side and slightly behind the centre. 3. The ball is brought back behind the head, then thrown as far as possible forward. 4. The athlete is allowed to step forward once the ball has been released and this is part of the throwing technique for maximal distance and power. 5. Repeat the test three times. 6. The assistant uses the longest of the three throws as the final result.

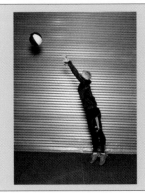

Target scores

	Female		Male	
	Junior	Adult	Junior	Adult
Excellent	6.90m+	7m+	9.30m+	10m+
Good	5.75–6.90m	5.90–7m	7.80–9.30m	8.85–10m
Average	4.25–5.75m	4.60–5.90m	6.10–7.80m	7–8.85m
More training required	<4.25m	<4.60m	<6.10m	<7m

Table 136   Target scores for medicine ball throw.

Overhead Reverse Medicine Ball Throw

This test is the reverse action of the forward medicine ball throw. You should always use the same weight medicine ball either a 2kg or 5kg, depending on the age and experience of the person being tested. As with the forward throw, there is an optimal release high point that needs to be coached and learned correctly before this test is considered a useful tool.

Equipment
<ul><li>Medicine ball</li><li>Tape measure</li><li>Assistant</li></ul>
Procedure
1. The athlete follows a pre-described warm-up protocol. 2. The athlete stands in an athletic position with heels touching the start line. The medicine ball is held above the head with hands on the side and slightly behind the centre. 3. The ball is lowered to hip height in front of the athlete and then moved rapidly upwards above and behind the head to be thrown as far as possible backwards. 4. The athlete is allowed to step backwards once the ball has been released and this is part of the throwing technique for maximal distance and power. 5. Repeat the test three times. 6. The assistant uses the longest of the three throws as the final result.

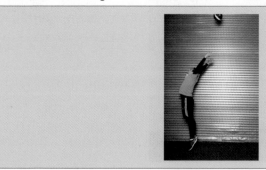

Target scores

	Female		Male	
	Junior	Adult	Junior	Adult
Excellent	9.90m	10.50m	13.5m	14m
Good	8–9.90m	8.20–10.50m	10.50–13.50m	11.50–14m
Average	6.50–8m	6–8.20m	8.50–10.50m	9.50–11.50m
More training required	<6.50m	<6m	<8.50m	<9.50m

Table 137   Target scores for overhead reverse medicine ball throw.

INTERPRETING YOUR DATA

All these tests are useful when comparing previous data for the athlete being tested. The counter-movement jump is what most people refer to when they are stating how high they can jump and, along with the static vertical jump, can be a useful tool in determining the effectiveness of the stretch-shortening cycle. An athlete's score for his or her counter-movement jump should be approximately 15 per cent more than the static vertical jump. If your score is less than this you should consider following a progressive maximal strength-related programme, as detailed in Chapter 4.

Your running vertical jump should be both higher than your static and counter movement jump scores, which makes perfect sense due to the increased momentum and stretch-shortening cycle action prior to take-off.

Technique is the key to any testing performance score and adequate time should be spent teaching the technique required for optimal testing results. Arm swings can add an additional 15 to 20 per cent on jump height scores and should therefore be practised before undertaking test procedures.

Upper body tests requiring throws should use the appropriate medicine ball for the athlete, which allows for sound technique. Increases in med ball weight should be seen as a progression rather than a necessity by both athlete and coach. Remember that correct technique and practice should always be the premise of any athlete or coach and using a med ball that is too heavy will not only increase the propensity to injury but also discourage the athlete with what they consider to be sub-maximal performances.

Depending on the equipment that you use for collecting your results, it can be useful to collect power scores. If you are using the methods described above that use simple 'chalk and measure' test procedures then you can use some simple equations to work out a power score. While the purpose of a jump test is to look at absolute results such as a jump height achieved, it is sometimes useful to consider that a heavier person jumping the same height as somebody lighter than them is actually exerting more power.

In these test protocols, power cannot be calculated accurately since time cannot be measured accurately unless you are using a jump mat (remember Power = Work ÷ Time). If you are fortunate to have equipment such as a jump mat or Tendo unit that can measure one or all of the variables then, fantastic, they will give you a power reading for your test. For most of us though this will not be the case and many formulae have been developed for estimating power for vertical jump measurements. I sometimes use the calculations shown in Fig. 9.2 to calculate peak and average power.

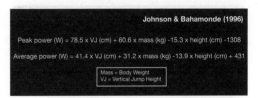

Johnson & Bahamonde (1996)

Peak power (W) = 78.5 x VJ (cm) + 60.6 x mass (kg) -15.3 x height (cm) -1308

Average power (W) = 41.4 x VJ (cm) + 31.2 x mass (kg) -13.9 x height (cm) + 431

Mass = Body Weight
VJ = Vertical Jump Height

Fig 9.2 Calculating peak and average power. (Source: Johnson and Bahamonde, 1996)

OTHER TEST OPTIONS

Any plyometric movement can be used as a test as long as it follows the principles described at the beginning of this chapter. An additional method often used by coaches is the pentathlon, heptathlon or decathlon plyometric competition. Athletes perform five, seven or ten separate plyometric tests involving single or multiple movements such as the standing long jump, single hops, multiple two or single foot jumps or combination jumps, as well as med ball throws. These are generally measured for distance with a descending points scale given for those athletes who come first to last in the test group in each event. These can be great fun and very motivating sessions for both athletes and coaches, while also counting as a training session in their own right.

Index

160